Herbal Apothecary:
Top 150 Medicinal Herbs For Healthy Living and Healing

Table of content

Introduction: The Best Things Come from Scratch!

About as far back as conscious, human recollection goes, herbs from man's natural environment have been used for medicinal purposes. They were used in India over 5000 years ago in the form of Ayurvedic Medicine. And in ancient Greece, for a physician named Aristotle, the power of flowers, fruits, seeds and roots, was just what the doctor ordered.

Herbal medicine was the standard form of treatment for much of the world for centuries. In the past when someone was sick they would pay a visit to their local herbal expert who would find just the right ingredient to help them. A sorely missed ingredient for most of us in modern life, since in much of the prepackaged and mass produced modern world, we are hard pressed to even find herbs in the food we eat, let alone are medicine. But as this book bears testament—things are starting to change!

And herbal therapies are starting to make a major come back. And one of the most popular herbal therapies to make some headway is that of Aromatherapy. With its roots firmly affixed to the incense burners of the ancient world, this herbal practice has us purposefully inhaling the fragrance of specific herbs in order to create a desired reaction in our body. A powerful treatment that has now sprung up as special Aromatherapy clinics attached to many major hospitals.

In recent years the use of taking the essential oils from medicinal herbs and using them in specifically targeted massage therapy has also become in vogue. We will discuss both of these practices and many more methods further in this book. For right now I just want to captivate your imagination with the possibilities and ignite your awareness of the impact that these powerful medicinal herbs can have on your life.

Sometimes known as holistic medicine, medicinal herbs are used to treat the whole body. This holistic approach is something that modern medicine often lacks. Because often enough, when we turn to pharmaceuticals we find ourselves just masking chronic symptoms, whereas many herbal medicines are able to target the actual deficiency itself, which is the source of the problem. Showing once again that, most of our aches and pains are simply our body crying out for something that it lacks.

Because when you break it all down, just as the Christian/Hebrew bible and many other ancient religious traditions remind us; we came from the dust of the Earth. We truly are part and parcel to this planet, and all of the molecules, all of the proteins, amino acids and other trace elements in our body can be found strewn all over the Earth. So if this is from whence we came, and we find that our body is lacking something, all we have to do is look to the Earth to find it. We don't need to replicate and synthesize chemicals in a pharmacy; all we have to do is look to nature and the medicines that it naturally provides. Because the best things truly do come from scratch!

Chapter 1: Aromatherapy; A Nose above the Rest!

The human nose is an intricate piece of sensory machinery, we may not be aware of the complexities involved in smelling a cup of coffee, but that doesn't mean that they are not there. Called the "Chemosensory System" the nose is part of a joint apparatus that works to use the senses of taste and smell in order to help us interpret our environment.

For thousands of years our sense of smell has served to help us find a meal, tell us of potential threats, and through pheromones that trigger powerful chemosensory responses, has even played a role in determining our mates. We may take it for granted and not realize how influential are noses are, but just try to go a few days without it and you will quickly realize what you are missing.

Our noses work hard to interpret our environment, constantly labeling and cataloging a vast multitude of chemical molecules that we inhale every time we breathe in the air. In an instant our nose is able to pick up the distinct chemical trace element of a campfire and then send it to our brain which instantly relates to us our fond memories of when we used to go camping with our Uncle Bernie.

Every time we smell a specific "smell" it is due to the fact that an odor molecule has bonded to one of the millions of "olfactory receptors" in our nasal cavity whose job is to interpret what those odor molecules are. Telling us whether something is bitter, salty, sweet, or one of a million variations in between. These incredibly complex interchanges happen in an instant—and faster than you can say, "This stinks!"—your nose is way ahead of you relaying that information!

As you can see, the nose is on the front line of our senses and working as a great interpreter of what is good for us, and what is not so good for us in the chemical makeup of our world. The nose also works as a natural gateway when it comes to the field of herbal medicine. It was also the original "gateway drug" in ancient religious practice in which incense was a common feature of inducing more mindful states for ceremonies and to relieve the stress of participants.

Frankincense

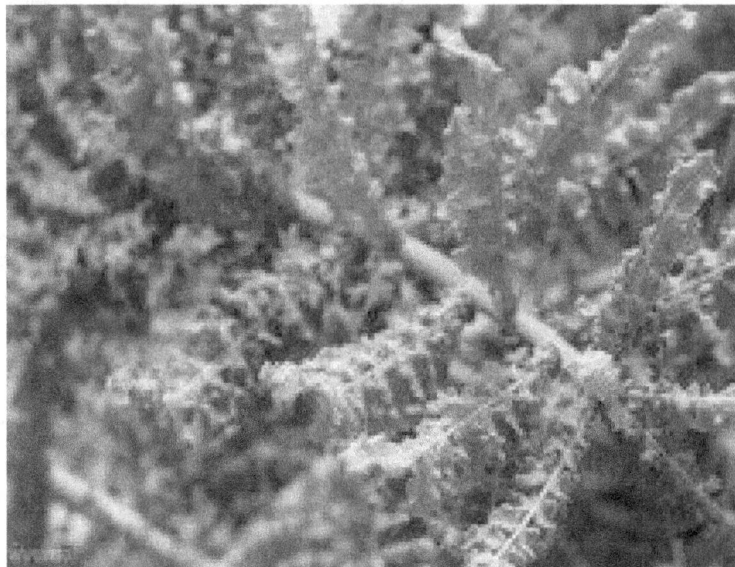

Powerful herbs were burned by the boatload in order to set the mood of the faithful. Smelling powerful incense was always a powerful part of religious service, making medicinal herbs a highly prized possession. And one of the most famous of these herbs is that of "Frankincense". Who could forget this wonder drug of the ancients? This was a medicinal herb that was so spectacular that it even made a cameo in the first Christmas story. Does anyone remember the three Magi who carried their Frankincense and Myrrh all the way from Persia?

In ancient times this stuff was of such high value that it was sometimes doled out as its own kind of currency. Frankincense was known to be able to alter the chemistry of the brain just by inhaling its fragrance. When the ancients were feeling a bit down in the doldrums they would just burn incense laced with Frankincense for an all natural herbal pick-me-up. And besides the elevation of mood it was discovered to have great affect on treating many kinds of inflammation.

It was quite a common practice for the local apothecary of yesteryear to either massage a bit of Frankincense into their patient's aching joints, or to have them just take a deep breath of their burning Frankincense cauldrons. Because just the smell of Frankincense alone can kick start a powerful chemical reaction in the body that cleanses it from impurities and boosts the immune system.

In modern day Ayurvedic circles Frankincense has even been known to fight cancer. Studies have shown that the application of Frankincense can reduce the onset or even reverse the incidence of Basil Cell Carcinoma (Skin Cancer), demonstrating exactly why this medicinal herb continues to be such a valuable commodity to this very day. Just by taking a breath of fresh air we can revitalize our entire system.

This is the basic premise that aromatherapy has been based on. But besides incense, one of the other traditional ways to take in the fragrance of medicinal herbs is to make an old fashioned poultice. A poultice is a distribution method of directly applying herbs to the skin, often around the neck and shoulders, so that the aroma of the herbs can be directly inhaled over a long period of time.

Poultices usually consist of dried out plant material rather than liquid and are crushed or mashed together and boiled with water before their application in order to make the ingredients more malleable so they can be easily pasted onto the skin. The poultice is often held onto the chest or neck area as a compress, fixed in place with heavy gauze.

Chamomile

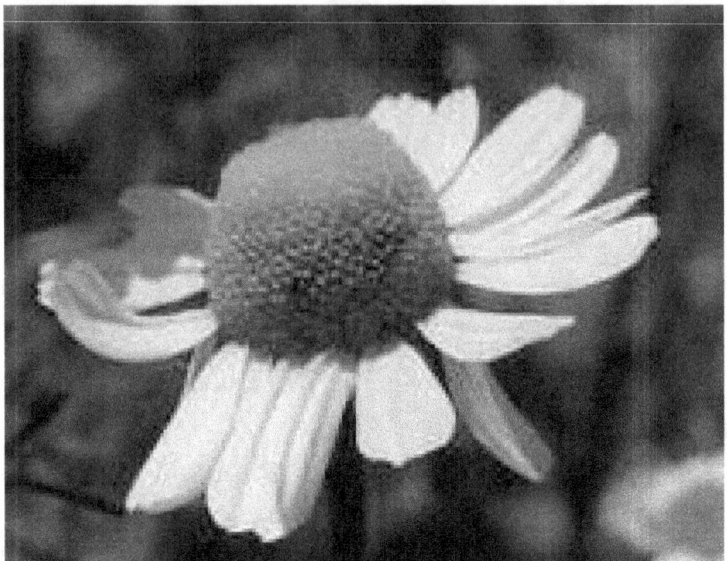

The herb Chamomile which is most famously known for its properties in tea also doubles as a great poultice. The crushed petals of the Chamomile flower compressed over a bruise or area of severe inflammation can bring immediate relief through this powerful poultice. The Chamomile poultice is also effective when placed on the jaw to relieve toothaches or around the ear to relieve a bad earache. But as mentioned you don't have to wear a poultice to get the effects of Chamomile.

Because a good strong blend of Chamomile tea can do wonders to alleviate muscle aches, as well as improve symptoms of anxiety and depression. And along with relaxing our nerves, breathing in the aroma of Chamomile has also been shown to relax our blood vessels, helping us to keep our blood pressure under control.

In order to get a good whiff of tea variety Chamomile make yourself a steaming hot mug and pour the tea into the mug hot. And before you even drink it, just put your face close and cup your hands around the mug and your nose, letting yourself breathe in deep the aroma of your tea. You can also just pull up a chair to your tea kettle and simply sit by the stove breathing in the steady aroma steaming out of your tea pot. Either way the effect is the same.

Bergamot

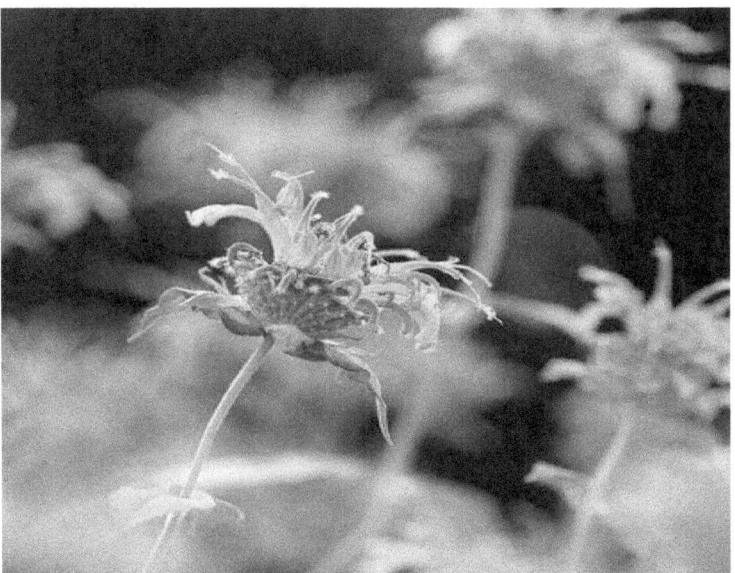

Very similar to the effects of Chamomile, is that of Bergamot, another relaxation inducing herb that can be used in either incense, a poultice wrap or in a great tasting cup of tea. Along with aiding relaxation, Bergamot has some other additional medicinal properties completely unique to this herb. With one of them being its amazing propensity to enable the body to completely neutralize the effects of fevers. Bergamot also works as a powerful disinfectant and antioxidant.

Due to its notable healing properties with the skin this herbal remedy is often taken with a bath either by placing a few drops of Bergamot essential oil (we will discuss essential oils further in the next chapter) or by specially manufactured soaps that have the Bergamot baked right in. Either way, with all of these powerful aromatic options, you will be head and shoulders (and head and nose) above the rest!

Chapter 2: Healing Through Essential Oils

Essential Oils are basically a refined gathering of plant based matter in liquid form. Inside this broad grouping of gathered plant material, we can break Essential Oils down into 8 main categories. They are; floral, citrus, herbaceous, spicy, resinous, earthy, and camphoraceous. All of these categories of Essential Oils are known to serve different purposes. But probably the most widely used however, are those that are derived from the floral family of essential oils.

Rose

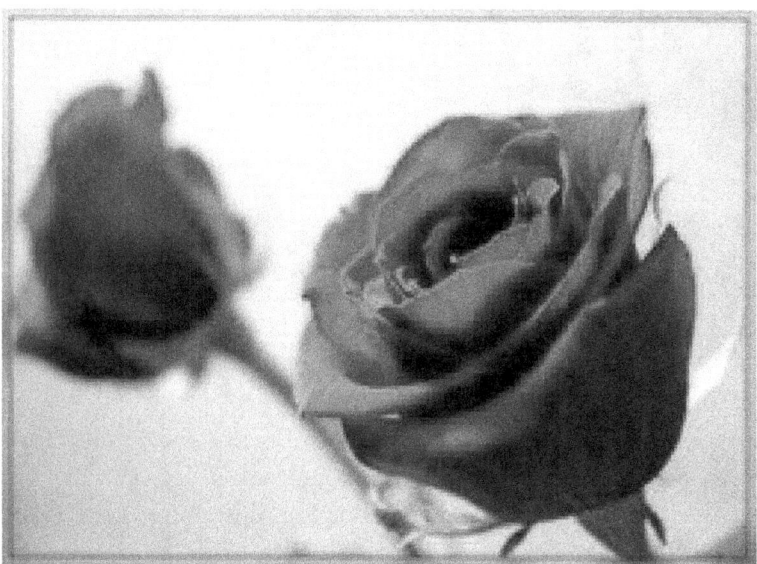

You don't have to look much farther than the expression, "It's time to stop and smell the roses." To realize just how widespread our attachment to floral fauna is. Roses in particular have been known to have many positive medicinal effects on the human body. For example, the petals from a rose when ground into essential oil have been known to be able to treat insomnia, stress, and depression. It has also been widely reported to be able to work as an anti-viral agent that helps boost the immune system.

Geranium

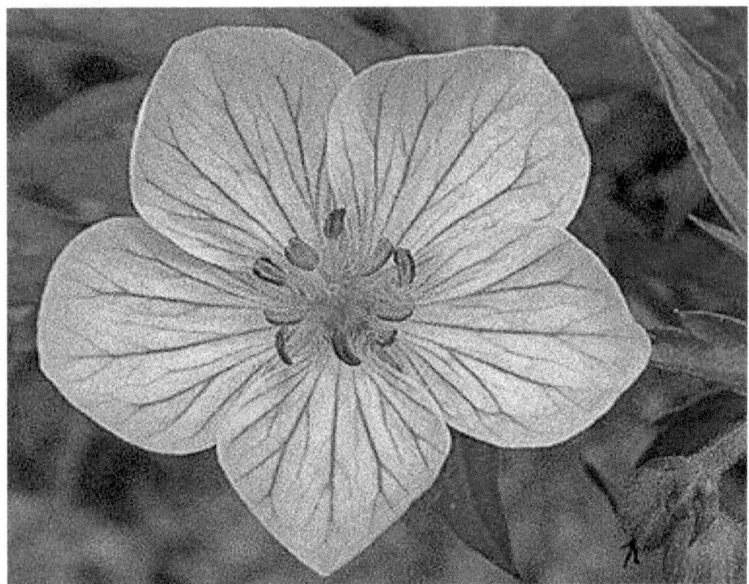

But as good as the rose is, it is also a costly herbal remedy, so much so, that many have opted to use its closest cousin instead. Because the oil derived from the Geranium is known to be nearly identical to oil derived from roses. Its benefits are also very similar, like roses the Geranium is known to have an immediate stress relieving quality when used in aromatherapy or when the oil is massaged into the skin.

Just like the roses, this essential oil also has powerful anti-viral and immune system boosting properties. Geranium oil also works extraordinarily well as a treatment for some of the side effects that women experience during their menstrual cycle as well as helping to alleviate the symptoms of menopause. Another reason that many women swear by this essential oil is also due to its widely known ability to reduce stretch marks which of course is a welcome relief after pregnancy.

But whether it is used for men or women, the compounds found in Geranium essential oil have been known to be able to completely balance out our hormones and help us function on a more even keel. Germanium as a relaxing agent helps to make our muscles contract, it aids our blood vessels in their constriction, and even works to loosen up digestive systems that are plagued with indigestion.

The other interesting thing about Geranium oil is that it is what we call in the world of aromatherapy, a "circulatory oil". This means that rather than releasing the chemical compounds directly upon exhalation—as is the case with other fragrances—the inhalation of Geranium sticks with us and instead of leaving when we breathe out, it goes straight to our blood where it continues to circulate in the body.

But even though we don't exhale the molecules out, they do have to leave the body eventually, and it is the method in which Geranium leaves us that creates another pleasant side effect. Geranium essential oil can only leave us when it is sweated out of the skin. Turning the user of this substance into a living, breathing air freshener, emitting the attractive scent of Geranium just from perspiring! This can have many medicinal uses for someone if they suffer from excessive body odor and it has been known to work as a treatment due to its great deodorizing effects.

Lotus

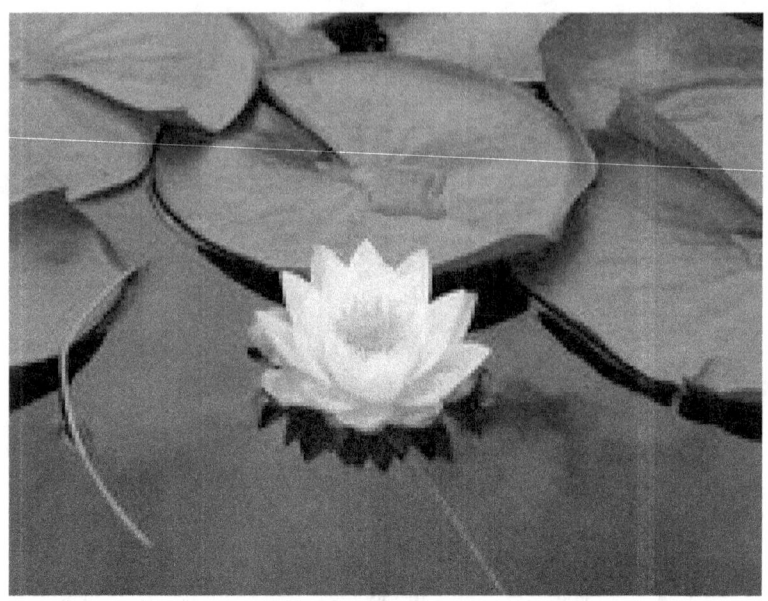

But probably one of the most celebrated oils to ever be extracted from a medicinal herb is that of Lotus oil. Known in the Eastern Hemisphere for thousands of years, the lotus blossom has been the stuff of legend. Along with countless Indian Yogi's down through the centuries, it is said that Buddha himself had prescribed this medicinal herb to his followers, making this medicinal herb a hallmark of two major religions.

But it is the essential oil extracted from this plant that can really create some mind blowing effects. Because just a little bit of lotus oil opens up the lungs and induces a feeling of calm. It would seem to be no coincidence then that the "lotus position" that has become so synonymous with Buddhism and meditation is associated with this flower. The lotus and its oil can have a major impact on our feelings of well being.

Jasmine

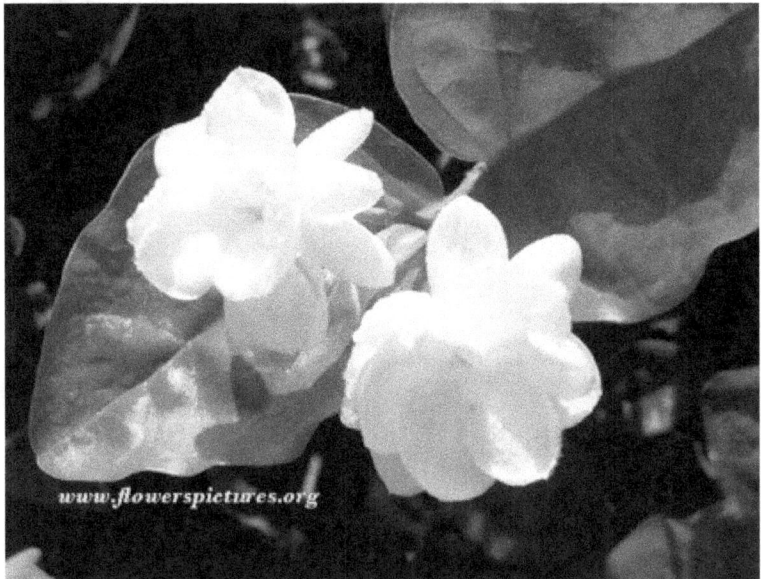

Right next to the effects of the oil from the Lotus, Jasmine essential oil is also a powerful medicinal herb in its own right. Coming from a flower that carries the moniker of "King of Flowers" the scent of Jasmine is unmistakable. I can testify about this from my own personal experience because years ago my senses were frequently inundated with this lovely sent in the most unlikely of places.

When I was still in college I used to do payroll for a truck company and right outside the door to our office someone had planted a ton of these Jasmine flowers and every spring when the flowers bloomed, we were all overwhelmed with their powerful scent. And whoever walked in the door when these flowers were nearby seemed to instantly perk up to their fragrance.

Even the big burly truck drivers who were on layover at our facility seemed to become rather pleasant and tranquil with this aroma around. Showing that even the toughest and gruffest of truck drivers need to take the time to smell the roses! Yet another example of just how soothing and medicinal the essential oils from these herbs can be; providing a bit of healing for us all.

Chapter 3: The Herbal Medicine Cabinet

Most of the time we are always hearing about the "latest" advances in medicine and high tech methods to treat illnesses. But what about some of the low tech options such as medicinal herbs that have been with us for thousands of years?

Because no matter what you may be up against, whatever sickness or ailment that you may be facing the immense bounty of nature and its medicinal herbs is bound to have the solution you are looking for. So let's stock up our low tech medicine cabinet on some of the most important medicinal herbs for daily health, as well as emergencies.

Echinacea

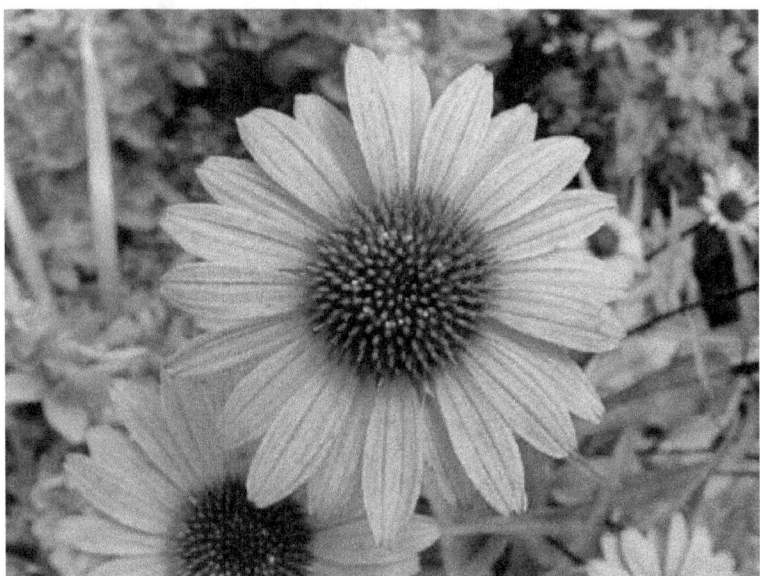

The first addition to our herbal medicine cabinet has been used by Native Americans for years for its anti-viral and anti-biotic properties. Echinacea is a potent herb and when ground into powder or the oil is extracted it is a powerful fighting agent against germs, viruses, bacteria, and even warts! So be sure to stock your herbal medicine cabinet with this precious resource.

Aloe Vera

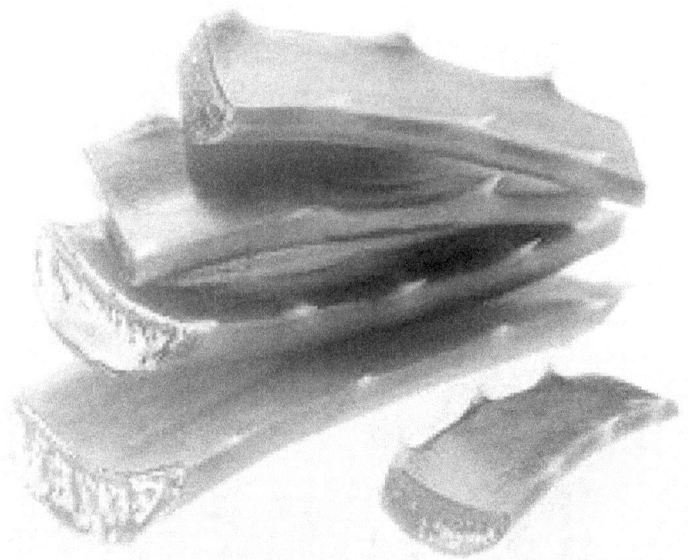

Growing up in Florida, as a child I learned from first hand experience that if you live in an environment with a lot of sunshine then Aloe Vera can be your best friend. Aloe Vera has been used to treat sunburns for a long time and is fast becoming standard fare even in burn units at hospitals. So if you are out in the sun and wind up with a bad burn it could help you out quite a bit if you have some of this stuff on hand.

Nowadays this Aloe Vera is fairly ubiquitous and you can find it at just about any CVS or Walgreens drugstore, but you don't have to buy it, because you can always just make your own. I'm a big fan of DIY and truly believe in the mantra that if you can do it yourself; then you might as well do it!

In order to make your own Aloe Vera you will need a leaf from the Aloe Vera Plant, the leaves of this plant are naturally full of the very same gel that you would buy at the drug store. So just take a leaf off this plant and either break it or cut it with a knife or scissors and squeeze the gel out into a small bowl.

After you've squeezed the gel into your bowl you can go ahead and scoop it out with a spoon or your fingers and apply it directly to your skin. Or if you would like to save it for later simply cover the bowl and put it in a cool and dry place such as a cabinet or possibly a first aid kit.

Catnip

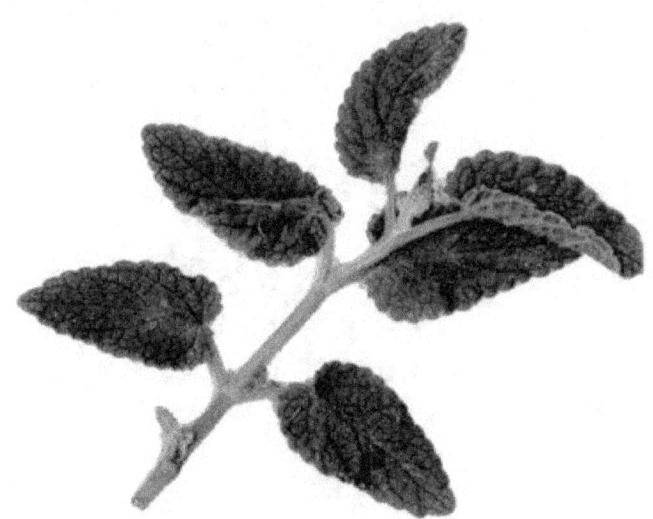

Our next recommendation for your low tech medicine cabinet is probably going to come as a bit of a surprise (for you and your cat) because as it turns out, catnip has many medicinal properties beyond making your feline friends go berserk. Catnip when used properly (for humans) is a natural cure for insomnia. Ground up leaves from the Catnip plant can be used to make medicinal teas that help sooth and relax those who drink them..

This same relaxing effect is also known to relax the digestive system, so if you are having stomach issues drinking a relaxing blend of catnip tea may be just the thing to put your troubled stomach at ease. It's also been well documented in its ability to help relieve headaches, so whether you are having trouble with your nerves, your sleep, your stomach or just have a nasty migraine, a medicinal blend of this catnip herb just might help you out.

Mistletoe

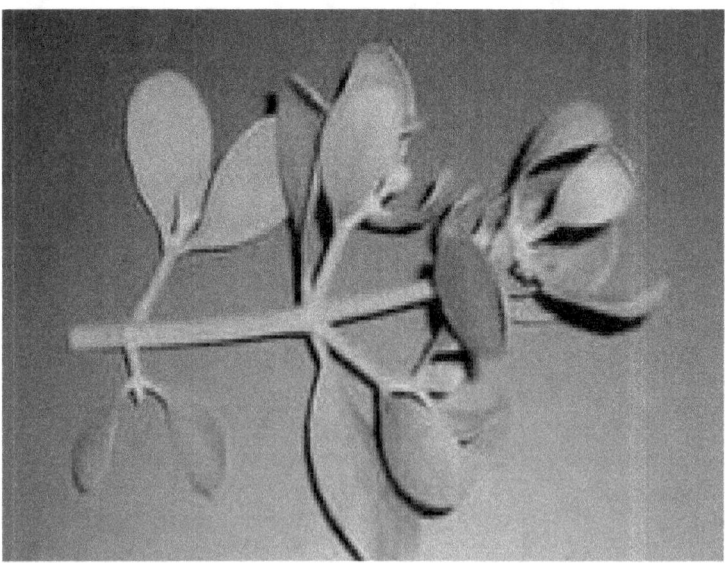

Another medicinal herb you may be surprised to find as a must have in your Herbal Medicine Cabinet is that of the most notorious hanger-on the holiday season has ever known; the Mistletoe. Yes, yes, I know you are probably rolling your eyes as you fight to keep "Ho, Ho, the Mistletoe!" from becoming stuck in your head, but please hear me out. Because this thing has a medicinal worth that goes far beyond holiday smooching.

For a plant that has such loving connotations, the Mistletoe's origins are actually that of a parasite. Normally found attached to Oak and Hawthorn trees, the Mistletoe receives its nourishment by leeching onto other plants. The great thing the Mistletoe does when it attaches itself to the nervous system of humans however, is that it has been found to be a wonderful anti-spasmodic agent that works well in treating convulsive nervous disorders such as epilepsy.

The leaves of this plant have been valued for quite a long time as a nervine and antispasmodic herbal medicine. In the past Mistletoe leaves have even been used to treat hysteria. Teas from Mistletoe leaves have also been known to help slow down a rapid heart rate, relieve high blood pressure, and soothe aching bones. But a word of caution however, the berries of this plant are mildly toxic and people have been known to get sick from eating them. The berries of the Mistletoe should be left alone; any medicinal properties of this plant should be derived from the leaves.

Garlic

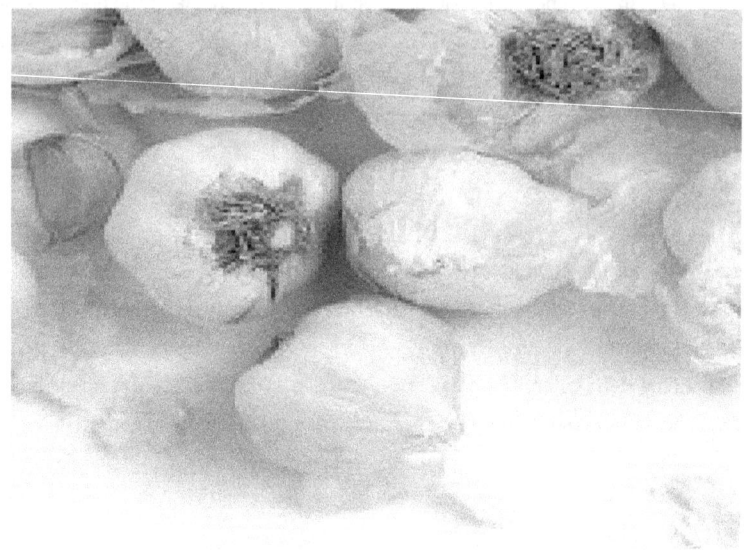

For the next installment in the herbal medicine cabinet we are going to suggest an herbal remedy that can work as an amazing antiseptic and immune booster as well as being rather tasty as a pizza topping. The herb I am talking about is Garlic. Known for its healing properties on the battlefields of the ancient world, crushed cloves of garlic applied directly to cuts and scrapes greatly speeds up the body's ability to heal its wounds.

Garlic is also known to be an incredible immune booster insulating the body well against colds and the flu, making this tasty medicinal herb a definite addition to the herbal medicine cabinet during the cold and flu season. This herb is best in its natural state, so keep a few cloves around that you can grind into powder or boil into your foods.

Astragalus

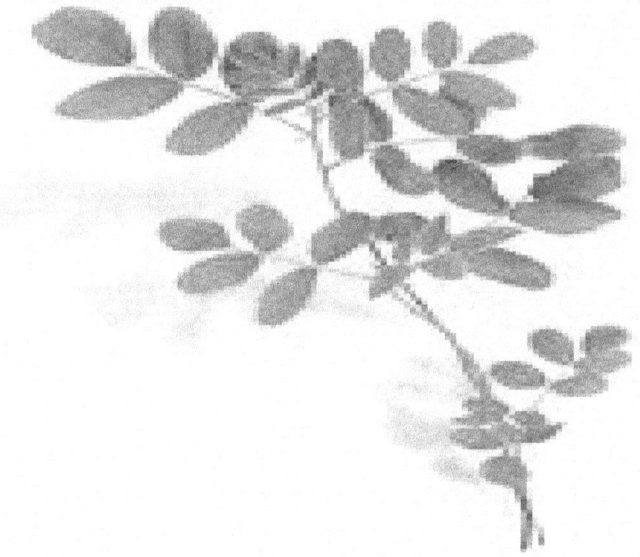

The Chinese herb Astragalus should be another addition to your herbal medicine cabinet. This herb has been used in Chinese medicine for years and is an excellent way to boost the immune system, fight colds, and energize the body. Astragalus is gathered as a root and usually ground into fine powder for use. It can either be applied directly to the skin or boiled in tea.

Dandelion

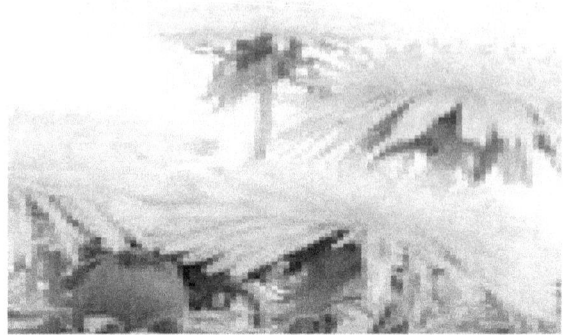

Although this herb is native to Europe it has become quite ubiquitous in North America as well. Known as the "backyard herbal remedy" in a real pinch the Dandelion can be quite useful. Dandelion roots can be drunk as a kind of tonic in teas and even "root" beers. The medicinal benefits of this magical root range from helping to aid indigestion all the way to promoting proper insulin function in diabetics. Providing powerful benefits for your health and making for a great addition to your Herbal Medicine Cabinet.

Ginger

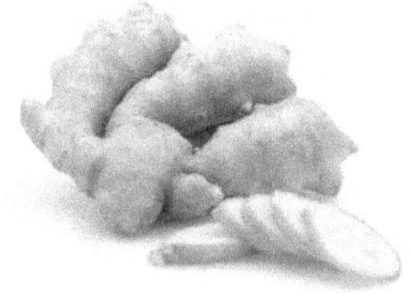

Ginger extract has been proven to have a positive effect on most joint and muscle pain. The main active agent within ginger that aids in this are called "phytochem-cials" an ingredient that works to lessen inflammation. Just grind ginger into powder and rub it into your aching joints for instant relief. You can also put into tasty teas and drink it for a powerful healing effect on your aches and pains.

Tumeric

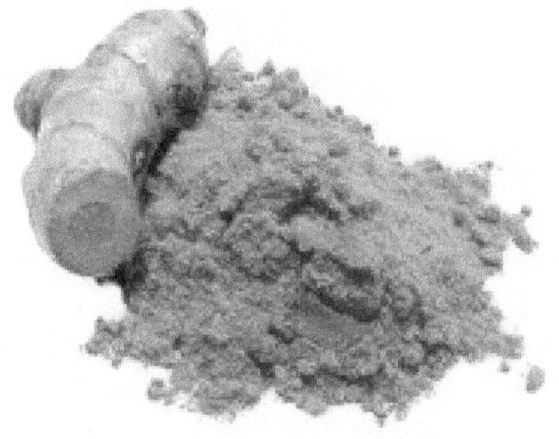

For those of you who suffer from chronic arthritis, Tumeric could be your best friend. Similar to Ginger, Tumeric works as a natural inflammation reducer. It's main ingredient "curcurmin" has powerful anti-inflammatory properties that ease their way right into arthritic wrists and joints. Tumeric is an ancient herb with a long history of practice.

Whatever aches and pains anyone has, Tumeric holds the promise to eliminate it. Along with arthritis Tumeric is also known to reduce heartburn, so whether you are suffering from a back ache or a stomach ache, it is still well worth a try. Tumeric is also a quite tasty seasoning for a wide variety of foods so don't be afraid to experiment with this pain neutralizing herb.

Devil's Claw

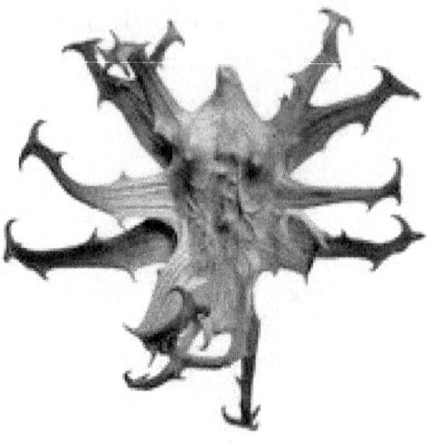

While this herb may not have a very appealing name, when it comes to the healing properties of this herb's, there is nothing devilish about it! Herbalists have used Devil's Claw to treat aches and pains for many generations. And for those that suffer from back aches in particular, this herb holds much promise. Because when Devil's Claw is ground into powder and applied in a compress to the lower back, it can provide great relief to back pain sufferers.

Hailing from South Africa this herb has been sought out from far and wide in order to avoid a visit to the chiropractor! And don't just take our word for it; there is documented research to back this up! In a controlled study in 2002 227 patients were administered this herb to treat back and hip pain, and out of these 227 patients, 70% of the participants reported improvement and even more than that an increase in mobility.

The active ingredients in this medicinal herb have the ability to loosen up even the most stubborn of joints and muscles to relieve your aches and pains. Devil's Claw can be found at most health food and herbal stores, and it can be grown for individual practice as well. So if you can get past this medicinal herb's strange name and appearance you will have a great asset on your hands when it comes to the battle against aches and pains.

Valerian Root

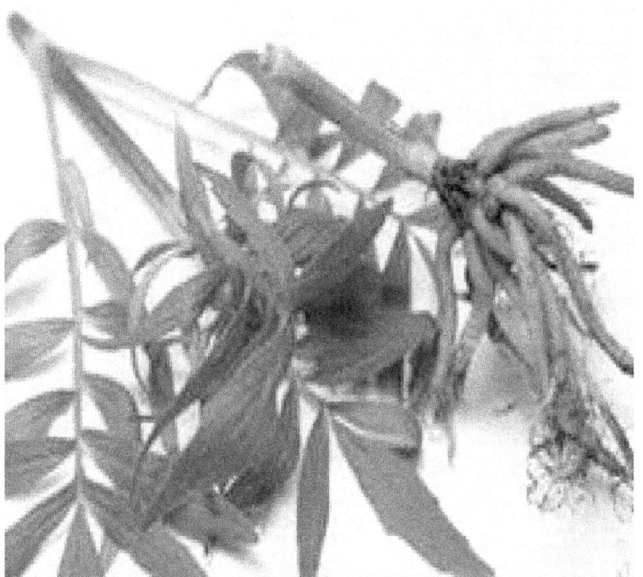

Valerian Root is a wonder herb and it has a long list of benefits, and one of the lesser known of these positives is the way in which this herb can relieve leg cramps and muscle spasms. Just apply this herb to the skin and let the soothing begin! Studies have shown that this root can work directly on the nervous system as a pain reliever. Valeria Root is popular for a wide range of musculoskeletal problems.

This root is also widespread, grown and found in large amounts in Europe, Mexico and India alike. Typical use of this herb involves either grinding it into powder, extracting essential oil from the root, or boiling the plant for use in beverages. I usually boil the root in a hot tea when I administer the herb to myself after a hectic day, allowing my aching muscles to relax!

Burdock Root

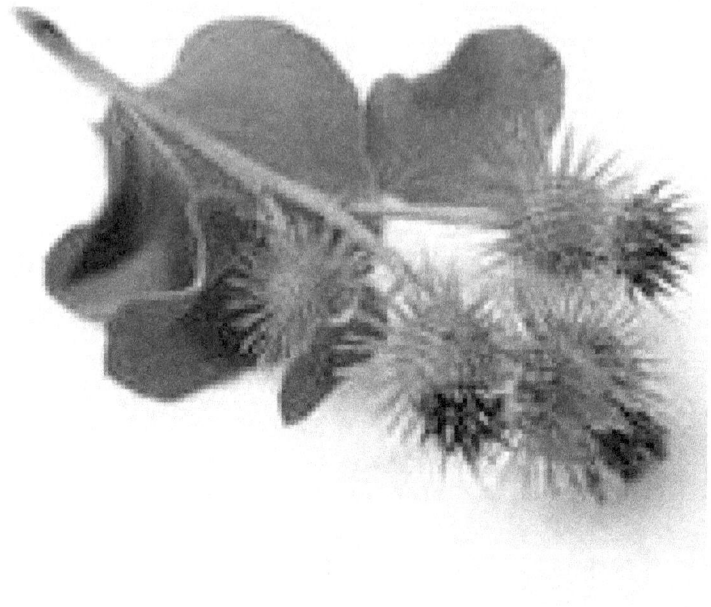

A dry and oily root that is known for lubricating and moistening even the stiffest of joints, Burdock is best used when ground into a fine paste or powder and applied directly to your aches and pains for maximum effect. The plant is easily recognizable by its wavy-edged, and arrow shaped leaves.

The flowers of the plant are usually purple or pink and appear in burr like clusters and can grow an astounding 2 meters tall. Burdock can be found scattered across northern climates all across the globe and is most prevalent in the late spring and early summer months.

The root of the Burdock plant can be ground into a powder and applied to the joints or a liquid can be extracted by boiling it. The essential oil extracted from this herb is very potent however so when attempting to use it just remember that old adage; a little dab will do you! You can use all of these great medicinal herbs to kick those pesky aches and pains straight to the curb!

Chapter 4: Herbal Aids for Weight Loss

With so many people suffering from expanding waist lines, in recent years we are flooded with a never ending litany of dieting fads and gimmicks. Carb restricting regimens such as Atkins and the Paleo diet in particular have become very popular as of late, but the only problem is, once you deviate away from these strict carb reducing regimens the weight comes right back.

The world of herbal medicine when it comes to weight loss has not been immune to criticisms either, as was most famously evidenced from the fallout Dr. Alan Hirsch faced a few years ago over his failed "Sensa" weight loss powder. Do you remember that? Sensa was a supposed aromatherapy based blend of aromatic crystals that people were told to sprinkle over their food to help them lose weight.

The jury still seems to be out on Dr. Hirsch's method, and if it actually worked, but when it comes to whether or not his clients had the right to sue him on false advertising, the jury emphatically agreed in the form of a 26 million dollar lawsuit. But what if we could bypass those mysterious "aromatic crystals" of Sensa and turn to a few proven herbal ingredients to enhance our diet and help to manage our weight the natural way? Look no further than "Rosemary".

Rosemary

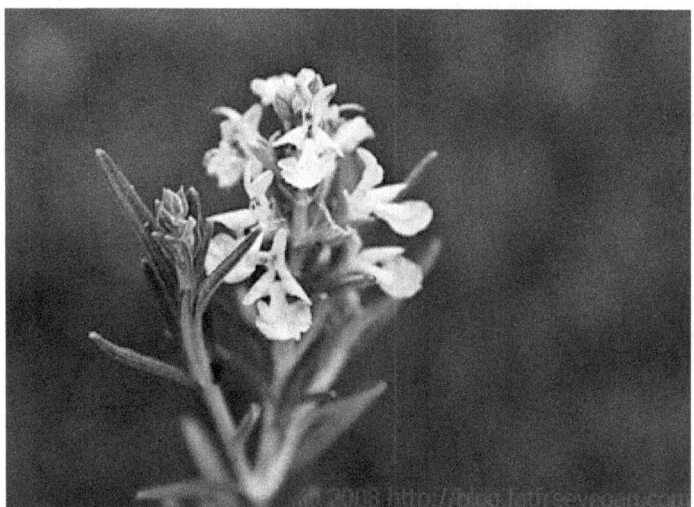

This medicinal herb hails from Asia and has been held in acclaim far and wide for its beneficial properties in regard to regulating weight gain and even eliminating cellulite. When this herb is consumed in a cup of tea it can raise your metabolism helping you to burn fat. Rosemary is also an excellent diuretic and the first weight that this herb will help you lose will undoubtedly be water weight, as this tea directly cleanses your system of excess water and other toxins.

After de-toxing like this, the Rosemary coursing through your system will bring you a new surge of energy and wellness; refreshing you as it cleanses. If you drink this tea for seven days straight your body will be primed, and streamlined with a higher metabolism and completely cleansed of toxins.

Rosemary works to eliminate any previous digestion problems, getting rid of bloating and helping you to break down food faster. As a result you will feel content with your food intake faster, curbing your appetite and keeping you from eating more. Most people lose at least a few pounds after their first weak of exposure to Rosemary and many more claim that this herb has toned their body and eliminated their unsightly cellulite.

Peppermint

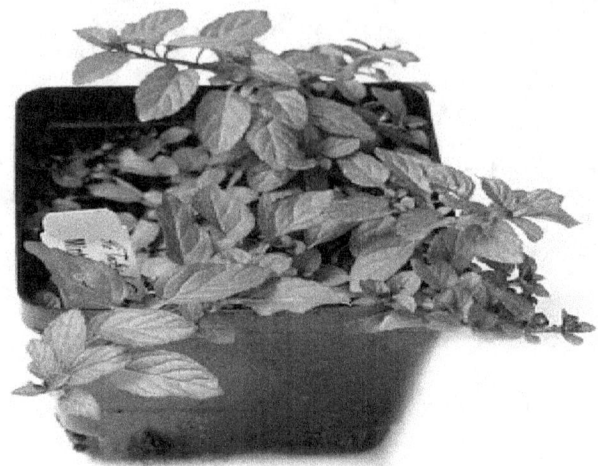

Another good herbal cleanser for the body is peppermint. Peppermint when inhaled and absorbed through the skin can directly influence bile secretion in the digestive tract. An action that helps to suppress appetite and further kick start your metabolism. Peppermint is best burned as incense and inhaled directly or even in a nice warm bath absorbing a diluted amount in your bathwater.

Ginseng

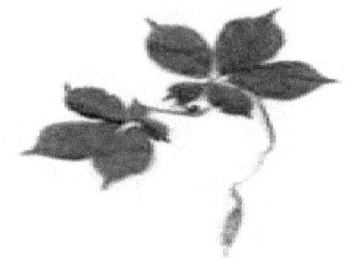

Last but certainly not least in our quest for herbal weight loss is the ancient Chinese herb of Ginseng. The roots from this herb are potent and have been known to boost the metabolism, but much more than this, Ginseng has the uncanny ability to alter the body's cells directly, altering their composition and actually rendering them less capable of storing fat. This herb and all the others mentioned in this chapter are most definitely welcome news for anyone seeking an herbal aid for weight loss.

Chapter 5: Herbs for Health, Beauty, and Cosmetics

Medicinal herbs can be a powerful force of healing in just about every aspect of our lives, beauty and cosmetics is yet another area where these natural remedies can apply. And if you are like 99.9% of the rest of the people on this planet, you probably tend to be a little bit concerned about your hair. Don't worry though because our herbs have us covered in that department as well. Because if you would like to have shiny healthy hair all you need is a few drops of a special little herb called "Sandalwood".

Sandalwood

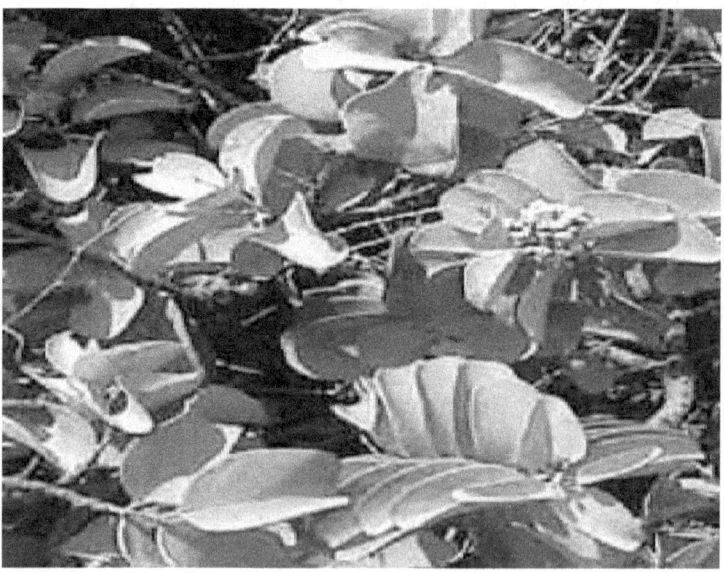

Sandalwood works as a powerful cleansing agent and along with shinier hair, sandalwood does a remarkable job of rejuvenating the skin and enhancing the user's overall complexion. Sandalwood can also work as an active ingredient in relieving the symptoms of Eczema and other skin disorders. Even better for those of us that have already sailed past the age of 30, Sandalwood is known to reduce the appearance of wrinkles. Sandalwood can work its way right under those bags under your eyes, reduce the moisture and make them disappear!

A great homemade mixture for Sandalwood skin cream involves one tablespoon of Sandalwood powder combined with a tablespoon of turmeric in about half a cup of water. Just apply this mixture as a paste to the skin and you will begin to see results right away. Let the paste dry off naturally and you will soon find that your skin has a clear and natural sheen.

Rosewood

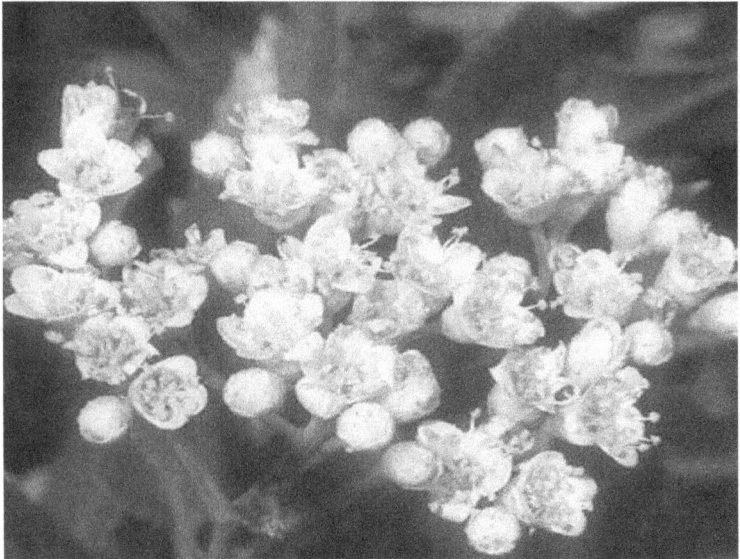

Rosewood is also a great herb for healthy skin and hair, and has been used in soap and shampoo since at least the early 1900's. Rosewood is extracted primarily from trees native to the great rainforests of South America, a fact that has unfortunately led to some pretty bad deforestation. Recent conservation legislation however has fought against this and the extraction of rosewood is highly regulated in order to prevent abuse and unnecessary waste of this precious resource.

Avocado

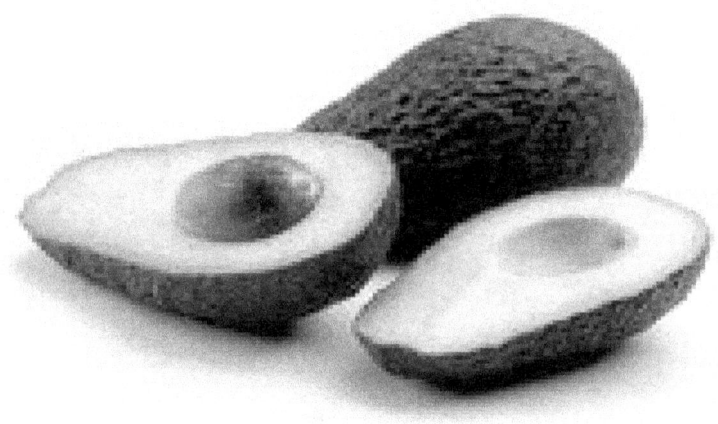

Our next notable mention for cosmetic enhancement you have probably used before to enhance your tacos! I'm talking about Avocados of course! Avocados have long played a role in that familiar face mask that many women (and some men) have ritually went to bed with over the years. It's sometimes remembered more as a running gag in TV sitcoms than as a viable health therapy, but a good Avocado moisturizer mask really can help your skin.

The active ingredient in an Avocado's oil is Vitamin D which works to penetrate and nourish the skin, helping to rejuvenate it and encouraging new tissue growth, allowing the surface level of our epidermal cells to stay younger longer. So if your wife ever scared you in the middle of the night by plastering her face up in so much bright green Avocado oil that you woke up thinking a space alien was in bed with you; don't get mad! Because the benefits of this medicinal treatment, and all of the others mentioned in this chapter, far outweigh the discomfort!

Chapter 6: Herbs for Fever and Cough

Items produced using botanicals, or plants that are utilized to treat ailments or to keep up the health are called herbal products, botanical items, or phytomedicines. Moreover, the item produced using plants and utilized exclusively for inside use is called a herbal supplement. Furthermore, numerous doctor prescribed medications and over-the-counter prescriptions are additionally produced using plant subsidiaries.

Home grown supplements come in all structures i.e., capsule, dried, powdered, or fluid, and can be utilized as a part of different ways, including:

- Gulped as pills

- Prepared as tea

- Rubbed to the skin as gels

- Added to shower water

The act of utilizing home grown supplements goes back a large number of years. Today, the utilization of home grown supplements is regular among American shoppers. Nonetheless, natural supplements are not for everybody. Since they are not subject to close examination by the FDA, or other representing organizations, the utilization of home grown supplements stays disputable. It is best to counsel your specialist about any indications or conditions you are encountering and to examine the utilization of home grown supplements.

How to cure fever

Many researchers have discovered homemade medicines using herbs and plants that can prove to be useful in curing fever. Some of the approaches that can be used to cure fever are as follow:

1. In order to avoid dehydration use of fluids to a large number is suggested. To flush the sickness away, herbal teas of following herbs are suggested

    - Chamomile

    - Catnip

    - Peppermint

2. Moreover, another way used involves the use of elderberries. Syrup is made out of these berries. This syrup, consequently, helps in curing the disease

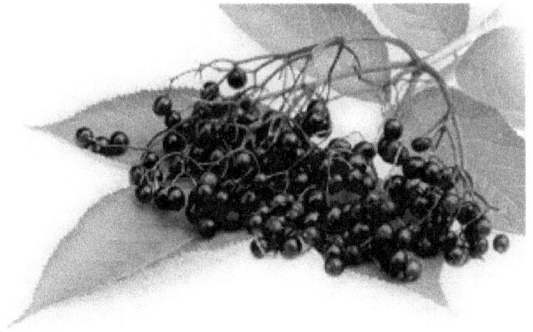

3. Mix some yarrow tea. Interestingly, this herb opens your pores and triggers the sweating that is said to move a fever toward its end. Steep a tablespoon of herb in some crisply bubbled water for 10 minutes. Let it be cooled. Then, drink a glass or two until you begin to sweat.

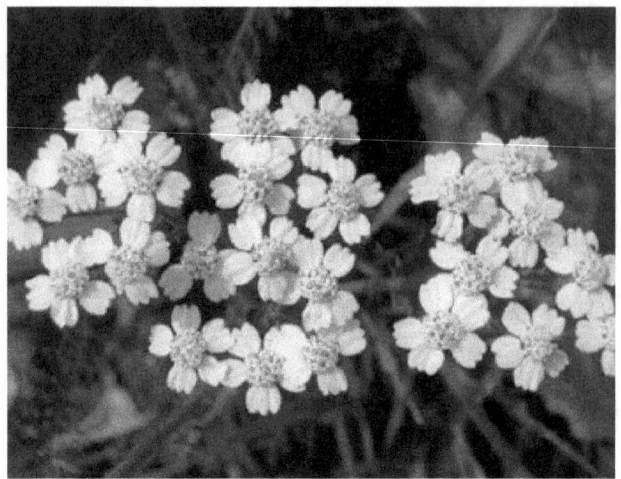

4. Another herb, elderflower, additionally helps you sweat. Additionally, it happens to be useful for different issues connected with influenza and colds, similar to overproduction of bodily fluid. So, to make elderflower tea, blend two teaspoons of the herb in some bubbled water and let it steep for 15 minutes. Strain out the elderflower. Drink three times each day the length of the fever proceeds.

5. Drink some hot ginger tea, which likewise actuates sweating. To make the tea, soak a half-teaspoon minced gingerroot in 1 glass simply boiled water. Strain, then drink.

6. Put some cayenne pepper on your food items whenever you have fever. One of its primary segments is capsaicin, the alarmingly hot fixing that is found in hot peppers. Cayenne makes you sweat furthermore advances fast blood course.

7. White willow has been utilized for a large number of years by Chinese doctors. A tea made of willow bark is maybe the best-known characteristic treatment for fever and torment. A dynamic compound is salicin, which was confined in 1830 and changed over to aspirin, a standout amongst the most well-known cutting edge drugs. The bitter taste of the willow Bark can be masked with cinnamon, ginger, chamomile, or any of various flavorful herbs

How to cure cold

Before the discovery of anti-biotic, homemade recipes were used in order to cure cold. In order to cure cold following remedial steps must be taken:

1. Get a lot of liquids. It separates your blockage, makes your throat soggy, and avoids dehydration in your body. The vast majority must drink at least ten to eight ounce glasses of liquid consistently.

2. You can relax up your stuffy nose while you take in some steam. Hold your head over a jar of boiling water and inhale gradually through your nose. However, care must be taken while you are inhaling steam. Try not to give the warmth a chance to harm your nose. You can likewise get some alleviation with a humidifier in your room. Moreover, attempt to take some relief from a hot shower.

3. Both saline spray and salt water are used in order to cure cold. In the event that you go the washing course, attempt this formula:

   i.   Blend approximately 3 teaspoons of iodide salt and 1 teaspoon of baking soda

ii.   Place the mixture in a sealed shut compartment.

iii. Now, add 1 teaspoon of the mixture in boiled or refined water.

iv.   Afterwards, fill a syringe with this arrangement and put your head over a bowl. Gently squirt the salt water into your nose. While doing this hold one nostril shut by applying light finger weight while squirting the blend into the other nostril.

v.   Let it deplete for some time and after a few moments treat the other nostril.

vi.   However, be very careful and make use of refined, sterile, or pre-boiled water when you make this arrangement. Or else you may catch a disease.

vii. Additionally, flush the globule after utilization and leave open to air dry.

Chapter 7: Herbal Antiseptics

Antiseptic herbs are an operator that slaughters or restrains the development of microorganisms on the outer surfaces of the body and are by and large recognized from natural anti-infection agents that decimate microorganisms inside.

A germicide when connected to wounds and diseases, guarantee that they are perfect and don't deteriorate and have been utilized all through history. A germicide is just a substance that can be put straightforwardly on a slice or contamination to guarantee that it is legitimately spotless and is going to stay perfect as could be expected under the circumstances until the following application.

Germ-killers avoid and balance contamination and the arrangement of discharge by repressing the development of the irresistible life forms. Germs are all around. Some take up habitation in our bodies and benefit us, for example, the amicable microorganisms that colonize the linings of the insides, upper respiratory tract, and lower urinary framework, out-contending terrible organisms, adding to invulnerable safeguard and great processing. Different organisms – infections, microbes, parasites – wreak ruin when they attack our bodies.

Luckily, various herbs have antimicrobial impacts. A considerable lot of these herbs are culinary herbs and flavors, for example, garlic, ginger, thyme, and cinnamon. That implies, regardless of where you will be, you can most likely locate a home grown partner at the neighborhood market. Herbs don't go about as fast or as intensely as medications. For genuine diseases, anti-microbial can spare lives. Then again, herbs produce fewer reactions and don't appear to be connected with the microbial resistance those diseases anti-infection agents.

Various herbs and oils are normal antibacterial and sterile operators and might be utilized as teas, skin washes, made into ointments. Clean herbs will be herbs that contain crucial oils are antibacterial and germ-free. For instance, Thyme is an Antiseptic herb that has been thought about and utilized since old times and the Thymol contained in the herb makes it an astounding germicide and antimicrobial. Numerous individuals are looking to reduce the impacts of artificially based germicides, on their bodies and there are numerous herbs and vital oils that have sterile properties.

Some of the herbal antiseptics that are useful and can help you in the wilderness are as follows:

Cranberry

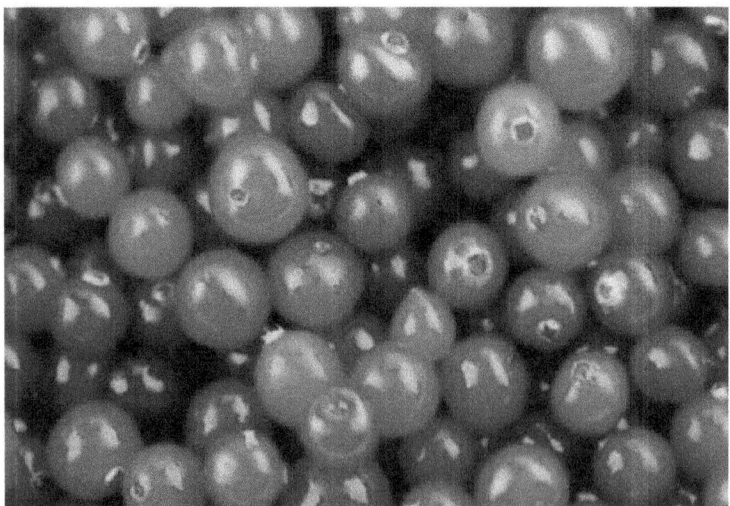

Cranberry also known as Vaccinium macrocarpon is taken as a juice or gathered in tablet structure. It meddles with bacterial adherence to bladder lining, accordingly averting disease. A large portion of the exploration has been in ladies mostly elderly ladies, youthful sexually-dynamic ladies, and pregnant ladies. They are inclined to rehash bladder contaminations. When disease starts, the microbes have effectively connected to the bladder lining. By then, anti-infection agents can clear the contamination quickly and keep microscopic organisms from climbing to the kidneys. For counteractive action, the juice dose utilized as a part of studies reaches from 4 to 32 ounces a day. On the other hand, concentrated juice concentrate can be taken at a dose of one 300-400 milligram tablet, a few times each day. Reactions can incorporate gastrointestinal bombshell. Likewise, concoction constituents of cranberry may hinder the proteins that separate medications, in these way raising blood levels of prescriptions, for instance

- Coumadin

- Valium

- Elavil

- Motrin, and others

Garlic

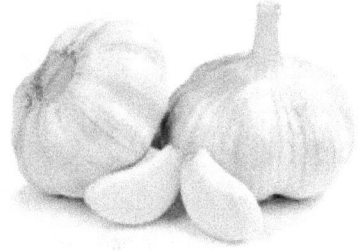

Garlic has antibacterial action against Staphylococcus, Streptococcus, Proteus, Pseudomonas, Mycobacterium, and in addition species connected with loose bowels. However, to some degree strangely, garlic meddles with sickness bringing about microscopic organisms, as opposed to the "amicable" microorganisms, for example, Lactobacillus that colonizes the digestion tracts.

Moreover, garlic is also useful in tackling various species of fungi. Antiviral movement incorporates influenza An and B, rhinovirus, cytomegalovirus, HIV, rotavirus, herpes simplex infection 1 and 2, and a few species that results in pneumonia. According to a particular research those people who use a garlic supplement commencing November through February had few chances of getting sick due to fewer than all those people who use pills. Other Allium types (chives, leeks, onions) have antimicrobial drive as well.

A significant part of the data related to garlic's antimicrobial strength instigates from lab ponders. A smaller amount is thought about in what manner garlic arrangements graft in people contaminated by means of these "bugs." The similar can be assumed in regards to the greater part of alternate herbs recorded beneath. Heat neutralizes garlic's antimicrobial elements. Therefore, it's preeminent to devour it crude or as a pill that promises a specific amount of allicin. On the off chance that you spread over garlic topically as an adhesive, ensure the skin using olive or any other type of oil, spread with dressing or clean material, and evacuate following 60 minutes.

Marshmallow root:

Marshmallow is most normally used to straightforwardness sore throats and dry hacks. The Marshmallow plant contains polysaccharides that have antitussive, adhesive, and antibacterial properties. In light of this, marshmallow soothingly affects aggravated films in the mouth and throat when ingested orally, particularly a sore throat. The antitussive properties diminish dry hacking and avoid further aggravation.

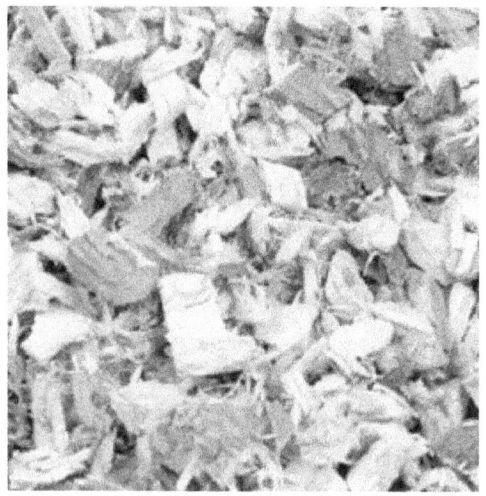

According to the research, marshmallow has been utilized to treat certain digestive issue, including acid reflux, heartburn, ulcerative colitis, stomach ulcers and Crohn's sickness. The system by which it calms sore throats applies to gastrointestinal mucosa too and consistent utilization of marshmallow can help with the agony of ulcerative colitis and Crohn's, and keep stomach ulcers from puncturing. Marshmallow concentrate is now and again added to creams and used to treat provocative skin conditions, for example, dermatitis and contact dermatitis. Extra uses are right now being explored. Marshmallow might be a useful guide to radiologic esophageal examination. There is conditional proof that marshmallow may likewise help with respiratory issue, for example, asthma. Scientists may soon test marshmallow as a characteristic contrasting option to glucose administration in diabetes.

Chapter 8: Common Ailments and Their Herbal Cures

As our way of life is getting techno-astute, we are moving far from nature. While we can't escape from nature since we are a piece of nature. What nature has put away in for us we have not yet completely discovered? This can irritate point with people. Certain European and Oriental nations have been investigating the utilization of herbs and has been by and by since the hundreds of years. Awesome work has been done which escaped the regular man's scope and information .With life on tech-course for each person in the 21st century human sufferings are turning out with various names .The essential herbs have the answer, the general key is no symptoms and powerful cures. The cures are in a state of harmony with nature which is the greatest in addition to point where no other drug can guarantee these actualities. The brilliant certainty is utilization of home grown medicines is autonomous of any age bunches.

Following are some of the common ailments along with their herbal cure are as follows:

Skin problems

1. **Burns:**

   i. **Honey:** This is particularly useful for serious smolders. It will stop disease, invigorate skin recovery and keep the blazed region sodden. Nectar is preferred for smolders over about every single medicinal intercession, notwithstanding for severe singeing.

   ii. **Prickly pear cactus pads:** Wear gloves to hold the cushions while utilizing a sharp blade to delicately filet the outside skin off the cushions. You will be left with disgusting, oval stack of plant matter. Place the cushions specifically on the smolder and wrap the injury. For sunburn, rub the cushions on the influenced region.

2. Cuts and scratches.

Each one of us experiences sharp edges may it is a paper cut or a knife cut, regularly again and again. Here's the way to handle the consequences.

i. **Wound powder:** My natively constructed wound powder stops the dying, dries out the injury, represses disease and empowers recuperating. I by and large utilize a gauze the primary day and afterward leave the injury open a while later

ii. **Honey:** Stop utilizing the injury powder following a couple days and switch to nectar. It's viable against all known medication safe microscopic organisms and truly speeds recuperating. Simply cover the injury with nectar, swathe, and change the dressing every day.

iii. **Wound balm:** Use a mix of berberine plants, Siberian elm bark, rosemary leaves, dark walnut bodies, comfrey root, oregano leaves, and dried thyme. Include a quarter-container each of the generally ground herbs to a preparing dish and blend. Spread the mix with around a quarter-inch olive oil, cover the dish, and prepare overnight in a stove on its most reduced warmth setting. In the morning, let the blend cool. Press out and afterward warm the oil. Blend in finely cleaved or ground beeswax — 2 ounces for each measure of mixed oil — and let melt. To check hardness, put a drop of treatment on a plate and hold up until the ointment cools. It ought to stay strong however dissolve following a second of preceding it with your finger.

3. Rashes:

Rashes come in numerous structures, so medications will shift. Here are a couple of them.

i. **For hives:** Put on a tincture of Echinacea angustifolia root topically, utilizing a cotton ball to regulate it to the influenced territories. Take a half-teaspoon of the tincture inside every hour or so also.

ii. **For toxic substance ivy:** Jewelweed balm is ideal. Great added substances are calendula blooms, chamomile blossoms and Siberian elm bark, all of which will calm skin. Include some other herbs you need, however utilize the ethereal parts of a jewelweed plant for half of the dried herbs by weight. At that point, take after the same procedure as above for making the injury treatment.

4. **Stings and chomps:**

Utilize thorny pear as you would for blazes or Echinacea as you would for hives.

Intestinal Upsets

1. **Loose bowels:**

Any firmly astringent plant will work for customary looseness of the bowels. Blackberry root, the primary standby utilized for millennia, is greatly compelling. Krameria root, more seasoned pine needles just pulled off the tree, and wild (Geranium maculatum) are all extremely supportive for direction. To utilize, generally slash or crush your preferred dried herb. Add 1 ounce to a quart jug that can take warmth, and load with boiling point water. Spread the invention and let it soak overnight (or for two hours in the event that you truly can hardly wait). Drink it all through the following day. Rehash as required.

2. **Gastric disorder:**

To begin, make juice of 1 beet, 1 bit of green cabbage (about the extent of a medium carrot), 3 carrots, 4 stalks of celery and 4 leaves of crisp plantain (Plantago spp.). Plantain is a typical plant you can generally discover developing in front yards, and is random to the banana of the same name. Cabbage and plantain are the most essential fixings; however they don't taste great without anyone else. Alternate fixings will enhance the taste while helping your adrenal organs, liver and insusceptible framework. Drink this squeeze each morning for breakfast, have cereal for lunch, and have whatever you need for supper. Touchy gut disorder will clear decently quickly on this regimen.

Chapter 9: Boost Your Immune System with Herbal Remedies

Our immune system is our most important tool of survival, without it we couldn't even step outside and face day. Just like in the famous movie, "The Bubble Boy" without our built in protection from contaminates, we would literally have to live in a bubble just to keep from being compromised.

Your immune system uses an army of white blood cells to stave off invasion by the harmful bacteria and viruses that we encounter on a daily basis. Any given day of the week your body produces about 1000 million white blood cells. Out of this main army of cells, highly specialized white blood cells of your immune system known as "Macrohages" literally go on patrol seeking and destroying any germs that enter your system.

It is through our Immune System's constant filtering and elimination of harmful elements that we can remain healthy. Having that said, wouldn't it be great if we could give our immune system a little jumpstart every now and then. Well my friends, then look no further than nature, because there are quite a few herbs that can play a pivotal role in our immune health.

Echinacea

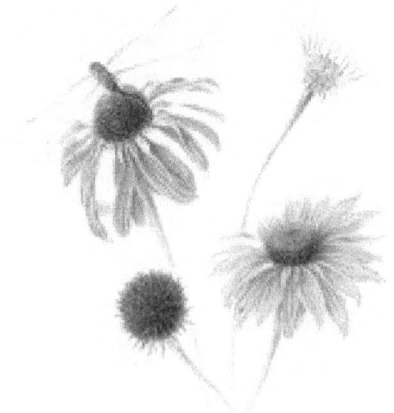

A member of the daisy family, this herb has astounding anti-biotic and even anti-viral properties and we would really be amiss not to mention it. Many herbal enthusiasts make a powerful tea and tonic from its extracted oil and use it to boost their immune system against bacteria, germs, and viruses. Just the aroma of this herb alone is enough to open the nasal passages. Moderate doses of this herb can treat even the worst cold and allergy symptoms as well as being beneficial to upper respiratory tract infections.

Reishi

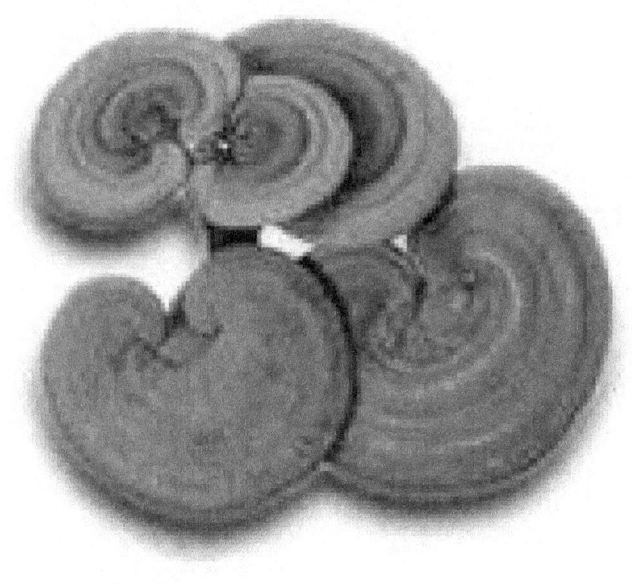

Also known as Ganoderma, Reishi is a bitter mushroom that has been used in Chinese herbal medicine for thousands of years. This herb has been shown to not only improve the immune system, but to improve longevity in general. Its heavy antioxidant properties have been used to treat everything from cancer to urinary tract infections.

Known as an "immune modulator" the properties of this magical mushroom work to fine tune and regulate your immune system. There is no special preparation required for this herbal remedy, really all you have to do is eat it and experience the results. In no time you will see that regular consumption of this herbal mushroom will improve blood flow and enhance your overall immune health.

Astragalus

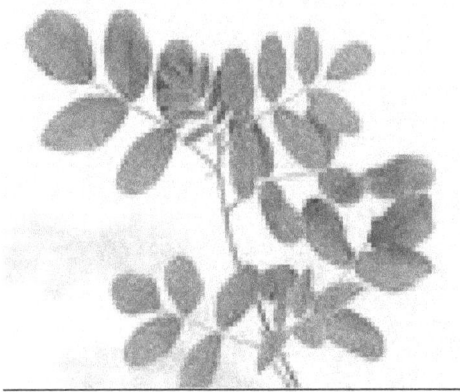

Another Chinese herb, Astragalus has been used in the Orient for thousands of years as herbal medicine. Sold by the boatload as dried root slices, this herb is still used to this very day as a powerful immune booster. Traditionally this herb has been served up in warm soups such as chicken broth.

An idea that seems to lend some credence to your mother's assertion that all a bad cold needs is a good bowl of chicken noodle soup! In fact as an immune system trigger, Astragalus has been found to be so powerful that it can directly activate the marrow of our lymph tissue and stimulate the development of our active immune cells.

These roots can be ground into powder and oil can be extracted to use in aroma therapy or as soothing creams for an herbal massage. The leaves of this plant can also be used to make teas that are good for the throat and empowering to the rest of our bodily function. This is an amazing herb and its benefits are well worth the trouble of obtaining it.

Cat's Claw

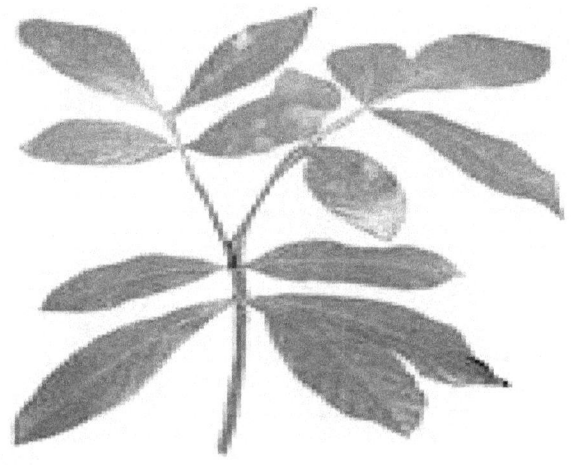

This woodsy vine is native to the rain forests of the Amazon in South America. Similar to the "Devil's Claw", the strange name of this herb comes from its somewhat odd appearance of curved, claw shaped thorns that look almost like a cat's claw. (If the shoe fits wear it right?)

But regardless of what it looks like the roots of this medicinal herb have been used for over 2000 years by the indigenous tribes of South America for their healing and immune boosting properties. When used properly this herb is known to significantly increase the white blood cell count and regulate the immune system.

These herbs have been recommended as an alternative therapy for both Aids and Cancer. For Cancer patients in particular, this herb has shown promise in helping to ease some of the harshness of chemotherapy. The root is typically served up in tea or ground into a powder that can be rubbed on the skin. All of the herbs mentioned in this chapter are all significant ways in which you can boost your immune system.

Chapter 10: Herbal Remedies for Anxiety and Depression

We live in a fast paced world, but unfortunately as we try our best to get ahead in our careers and social lives much of our peace of mind is left behind! In the hustle and bustle of the modern world we tend to neglect crucial aspects of wellness and stress free living.

And as a result much of the developed world, despite its technological progress, is in the full blown grip of anxiety and depression. And as stress levels rise millions of people around the globe are looking for new ways to relieve their sadness, worry, fears and frustration. But before you turn to more pharmaceutical meds, let's take a look at what nature can provide us to remedy our anxiety and depression.

Passionflower

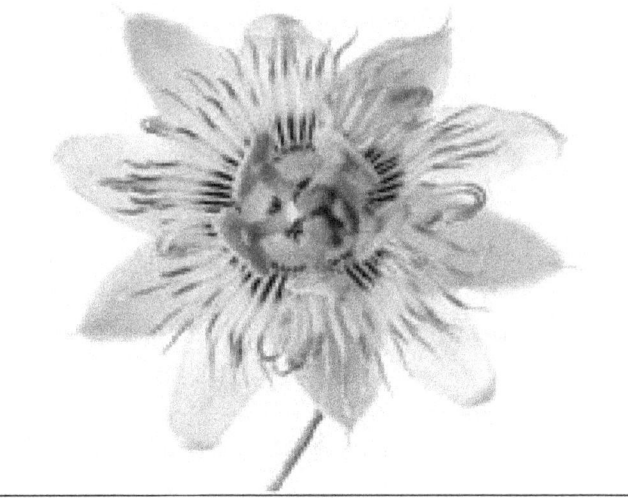

Once again demonstrating the power of the flower, this medicinal herb has been shown to work just as well as many pharmaceutical prescribed anxiety meds.

With its remarkable healing of depression, irritability, anxiety and agitation, this is certainly a flower to be passionate about.

You may have also have heard of passionflower as quite a popular beverage at your local star bucks. Yes just ask your barista, because they know full well that this flower most definitely has the power to make you feel pretty darn good!

Lavender

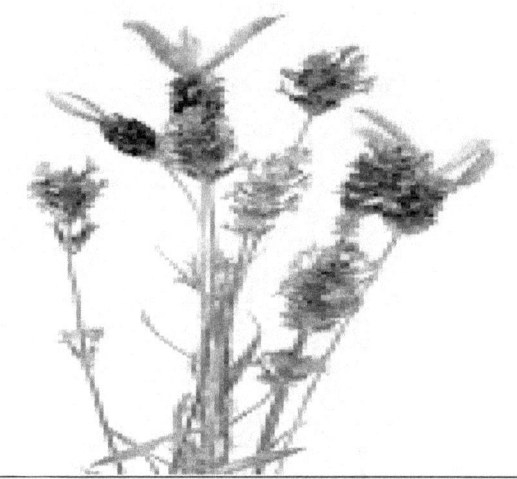

Lavender has been proven time and time again to be quite an effective agent against anxiety. An added bonus to this is that unlike other herbal treatments for anxiety such as Chamomile, Lavender does not have the side effect of making you sleepy.

There is no drowsiness reported from the ingestion of Lavender, so this herbal medicine can be taken at all hours of the day, allowing you to still stay alert and fresh. Lavender is often extracted as an essential oil and massaged into the skin or even worn as perfume, allowing its aromatic healing and stress relief to take full effect.

Kava

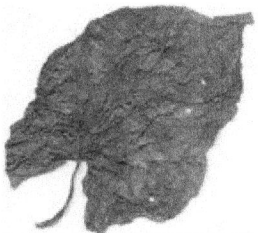

Kava, or as it is known in the islands; Kava! Kava! The Polynesians of the Pacific have used the roots of the Kava plant for thousands of years as a means to treat social anxiety. Viewed as a safer and less destructive version of alcohol, the boiled roots of this plant can be drank as an instantly relaxing tea.

Kava relaxes the body as a mild sedative but without interruption of cognitive function, so unlike alcohol you can relax with this herb without losing any control or quality of your everyday routine. Unlike alcohol Kava has not shown any addictive properties so use can easily be discontinued.

As great as some of the benefits of this medicinal herb are however, Kava is not without its controversy. And despite its proven benefit it's long term use has also been associated with liver damage, causing it to be banned in Europe. Kava is however still available in the United States at most health food and wellness shops.

Ashwagandha

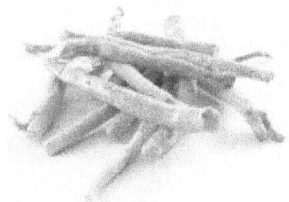

This medicinal herb has been a powerful part of Ayurdvedic medicine for centuries. Known as an "adaptogen" because of its ability to help the human body adapt, this herb gives you what you need to be able to get through stressful situations. The roots of this plant have a powerful effect on stress, gently soothing the body and the mind. The best way to take this herb is to boil the roots of it in teas and directly drink the benefit.

Lemon Balm

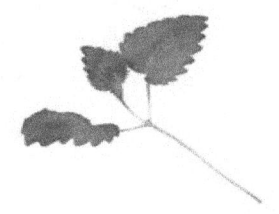

A medicinal herb from the Mint family, this herb has been shown to engender calmness for up to 6 hours after its use. This herb was used in the Middle Ages as a kind of tonic to reduce stress. It was a rather ubiquitous part of medieval society found in medicine, food, and even alcohol.

Today, this herb is still rather prevalent, and is used in many parts of the globe. It can often be found combined with Chamomile (another known calming agent) and boiled in teas and other soothing hot drinks. It is from the leaves that most of the medicinal aspect of this plant is derived.

The leaves can be applied directly to the skin as a cream or it can be reduced to a powder and absorbed through soothing baths. This herb is native Europe but can now be found growing just about anywhere in the world. The plant itself grows to about 2 feet high and is easily recognizable for its bright yellow flowers.

St. John's Wort

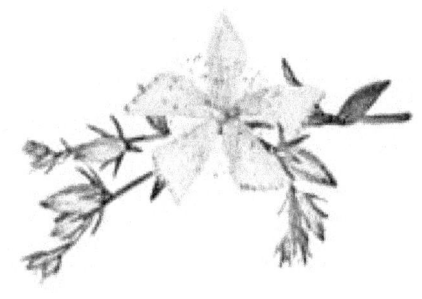

A friend had recommended this one to me years ago after my dad had passed away. She told me that it would help elevate my mood on the days that my grief had become too overwhelming. And while this obviously isn't a cure for grief in itself, it did help me out of the deepest aspects of depression.

St. Johns Wort is grown naturally in much of Europe, Asia, and North Africa. It has been used by Europeans especially to treat mod disturbances such as depression for quite some time. This herb has been associated with boosting Serotonin levels.

Serotonin is the body's "happy chemical" that directly bonds with the neurotransmitters of our brain to help make us feel good. Many people who have chronic depression suffer from a chemical imbalance in which they are lacking in this chemical. A medicinal herb like St. John's Wort helps to correct this imbalance and make you feel better.

Safron

This herb may not look too flashy, but it is a well known depression fighter. This plant is derived from the iris family and is found all over the globe. It is the end of the stem that is most often used to treat mild to moderate forms of depression. Safron is typically prepared by taking the strands of the plant and then either boiling them or grinding them into powder. Just sprinkle a little over your food or use it to make a relaxing tea. One great herbal remedy among many that will get you to feel right once again!

Chapter 11 – Perfect Plants for Any Plans

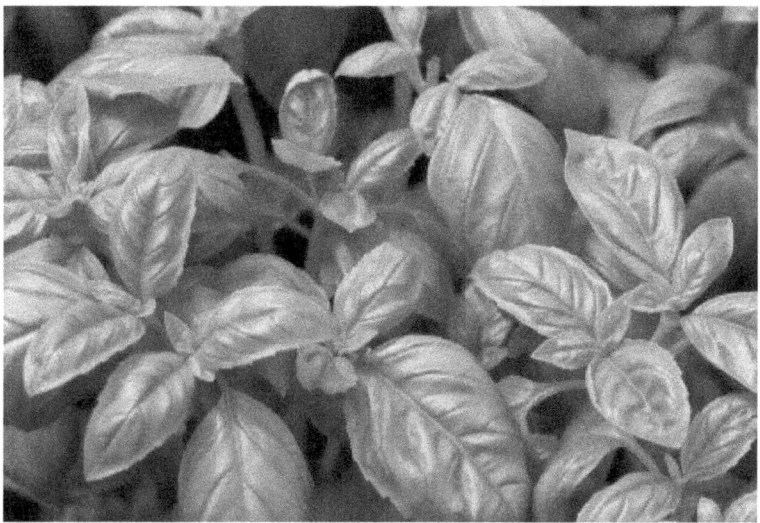

https://www.google.com/search?q=cilantro&source=lnms&tbm=isch&sa=X&ved=0ahUKEwi90e-gtLjOAhVXom-MKHT40BTgQ_AUICCgB&biw=1366&bih=623#imgrc=1UTsFkUdLSdQaM%3A

Lemon Balm

How to grow

Plant seeds sparingly in a pot, and keep in direct sunlight. Water morning and evening.

How to harvest and preserve

Simply grow your plant until they are mature. You will be able to see that they are by the way the leaves grow.

When they are fully developed and a uniform color, they are ready. Simply take your gardening scissors and snip off the leaves right at the base where they grow onto the stem.

Make sure you do not harm the stem as you work.

Lay them out on a paper towel to dry, or speed the process in a food dehydrator. When they are completely dried out, scoop the leaves into a small glass jar with an airtight lid until you are ready to use them.

Uses:

This plant has incredible calming effects. Use it to relax, calm anxiety, and soothe any fears.

Lemon Verbena

How to grow

Plant seeds sparingly in a pot, and keep in direct sunlight. Water morning and evening.

How to harvest and preserve

Simply grow your plant until they are mature. You will be able to see that they are by the way the leaves grow.

When they are fully developed and a uniform color, they are ready. Simply take your gardening scissors and snip off the leaves right at the base where they grow onto the stem.

Make sure you do not harm the stem as you work.

Lay them out on a paper towel to dry, or speed the process in a food dehydrator. When they are completely dried out, scoop the leaves into a small glass jar with an airtight lid until you are ready to use them.

Uses:

This is the plant to turn to if you are looking to lose weight and feel great. Anti inflammatory properties also make this a prime choice for swollen joints and pain.

Fennel

How to grow

Plant seeds sparingly in a pot, and keep in direct sunlight. Water morning and evening.

How to harvest and preserve

Simply grow your plant until they are mature. You will be able to see that they are by the way the leaves grow.

When they are fully developed and a uniform color, they are ready. Simply take your gardening scissors and snip off the leaves right at the base where they grow onto the stem.

Make sure you do not harm the stem as you work.

Lay them out on a paper towel to dry, or speed the process in a food dehydrator. When they are completely dried out, scoop the leaves into a small glass jar with an airtight lid until you are ready to use them.

Uses:

A member of the carrot family, this is a great herb to use for weight loss, healthy eyesight, and immunity.

Saint John's Wort

How to grow

Plant seeds sparingly in a pot, and keep in direct sunlight. Water morning and evening.

How to harvest and preserve

Simply grow your plant until they are mature. You will be able to see that they are by the way the leaves grow.

When they are fully developed and a uniform color, they are ready. Simply take your gardening scissors and snip off the leaves right at the base where they grow onto the stem.

Make sure you do not harm the stem as you work.

Lay them out on a paper towel to dry, or speed the process in a food dehydrator. When they are completely dried out, scoop the leaves into a small glass jar with an airtight lid until you are ready to use them.

Uses:

This could be considered the 'good mood' herb. Many people use Saint John's Wort as a natural form of an anti-depressant.

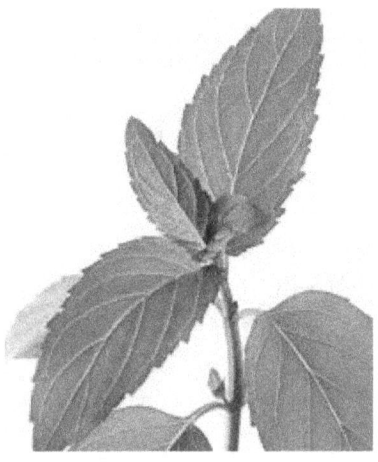

https://www.google.com/search?q=cilantro&source=lnms&tbm=isch&sa=X&ved=0ahUKEwi9oe-gtLjOAhVXom-MKHT40BTgQ_AUICCgB&biw=1366&bih=623#imgrc=1UTsFkUdLSdQaM%3A

Basil

How to grow

Plant seeds sparingly in a pot, and keep in direct sunlight. Water morning and evening.

How to harvest and preserve

Simply grow your plant until they are mature. You will be able to see that they are by the way the leaves grow.

When they are fully developed and a uniform color, they are ready. Simply take your gardening scissors and snip off the leaves right at the base where they grow onto the stem.

Make sure you do not harm the stem as you work.

Lay them out on a paper towel to dry, or speed the process in a food dehydrator. When they are completely dried out, scoop the leaves into a small glass jar with an airtight lid until you are ready to use them.

Uses:

Though this is an herb that is rich in flavor and can be used for a variety of health benefits including anti-inflammatory.

Chapter 12– From the Garden to the Table

Parsley

How to grow

Section plants roughly 1 inch apart in your pot, and place in a sunny area. Water daily.

How to harvest and preserve

Simply grow your plant until they are mature. You will be able to see that they are by the way the leaves grow.

When they are fully developed and a uniform color, they are ready. Simply take your gardening scissors and snip off the leaves right at the base where they grow onto the stem.

Make sure you do not harm the stem as you work.

Lay them out on a paper towel to dry, or speed the process in a food dehydrator. When they are completely dried out, scoop the leaves into a small glass jar with an airtight lid until you are ready to use them.

Uses:

Full of antioxidants, this is the perfect herb to use for all over health. By using this herb frequently, you are going to have an overall feeling of health and wellness.

Parsley is an excellent source of folic acid, meaning it is one of the best things you can consume for your heart. Not only that, but it is another excellent herb to include in your diet if you want to lose weight.

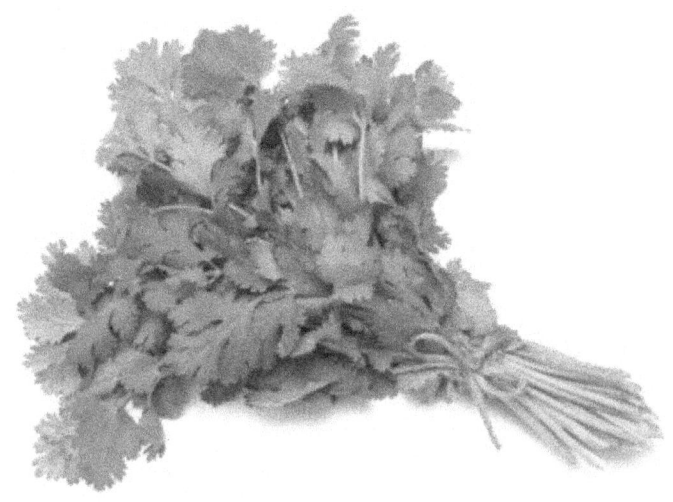

Cilantro

How to grow

Section plants roughly 1 inch apart in your pot, and place in a sunny area. Water daily.

How to harvest and preserve

Simply grow your plant until they are mature. You will be able to see that they are by the way the leaves grow.

When they are fully developed and a uniform color, they are ready. Simply take your gardening scissors and snip off the leaves right at the base where they grow onto the stem.

Make sure you do not harm the stem as you work.

Lay them out on a paper towel to dry, or speed the process in a food dehydrator. When they are completely dried out, scoop the leaves into a small glass jar with an airtight lid until you are ready to use them.

Uses:

Choose this herb for all of your cholesterol needs, and be ready to embrace the antioxidants that run abundantly through the leaves. This is the herb to turn to for excellent blood health.

Oregano

How to grow

Section plants roughly 1 inch apart in your pot, and place in a sunny area. Water daily.

How to harvest and preserve

Simply grow your plant until they are mature. You will be able to see that they are by the way the leaves grow.

When they are fully developed and a uniform color, they are ready. Simply take your gardening scissors and snip off the leaves right at the base where they grow onto the stem.

Make sure you do not harm the stem as you work.

Lay them out on a paper towel to dry, or speed the process in a food dehydrator. When they are completely dried out, scoop the leaves into a small glass jar with an airtight lid until you are ready to use them.

Uses:

This is a plant that is rich in vitamin K. Potassium and antioxidants are also found here, making this not only a great herb to cook with for the taste, but one you should choose for the health benefits as well.

Chives

How to grow

Section plants roughly 1 inch apart in your pot, and place in a sunny area. Water daily.

How to harvest and preserve

Simply grow your plant until they are mature. You will be able to see that they are by the way the leaves grow.

When they are fully developed and a uniform color, they are ready. Simply take your gardening scissors and snip off the leaves right at the base where they grow onto the stem.

Make sure you do not harm the stem as you work.

Lay them out on a paper towel to dry, or speed the process in a food dehydrator. When they are completely dried out, scoop the leaves into a small glass jar with an airtight lid until you are ready to use them.

Uses:

I could spend an entire day explaining all of the excellent benefits of chives. They are great for your circulatory system perhaps most importantly, and they are rich in vitamins.

Include in your diet often for maximum results.

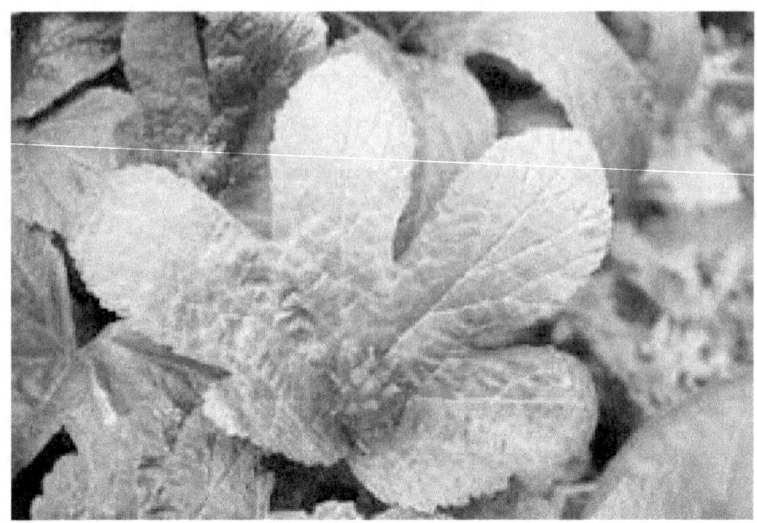

https://www.google.com/search?q=cilantro&source=lnms&tbm=isch&sa=X&ved=0ahUKEwi9oe-gtLjOAhVXom-MKHT40BTgQ_AUICCgB&biw=1366&bih=623#imgrc=1UTsFkUdLSdQaM%3A

Goldenseal

How to grow

Section plants roughly 1 inch apart in your pot, and place in a sunny area. Water daily.

How to harvest and preserve

Simply grow your plant until they are mature. You will be able to see that they are by the way the leaves grow.

When they are fully developed and a uniform color, they are ready. Simply take your gardening scissors and snip off the leaves right at the base where they grow onto the stem.

Make sure you do not harm the stem as you work.

Lay them out on a paper towel to dry, or speed the process in a food dehydrator. When they are completely dried out, scoop the leaves into a small glass jar with an airtight lid until you are ready to use them.

Uses:

In this modern world we live in, I can't say enough good things about a plant that fights cancer, and not only does this plant help prevent cancer cells from forming, it is also effective in fighting the illness.

Chapter 13 – Minty Madness

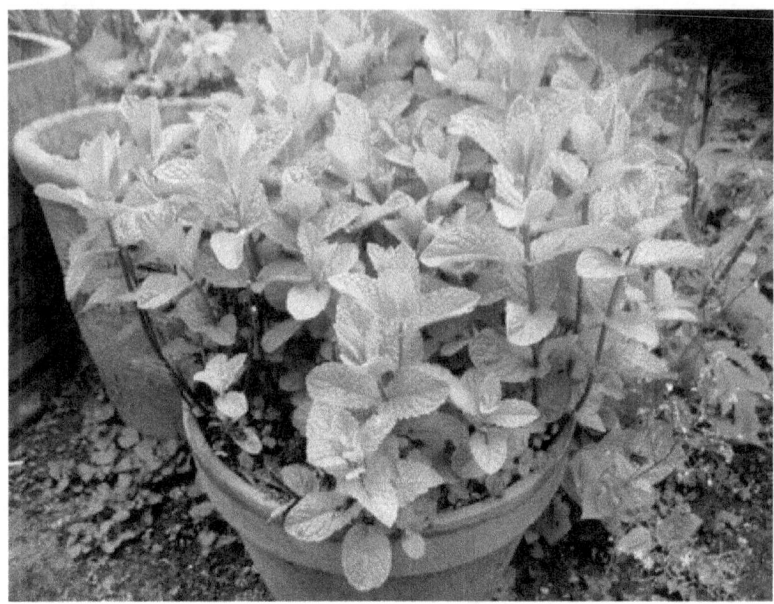

Peppermint

How to grow

Mints in general are really easy to grow. Place in a pot and leave in direct sunlight, water daily.

How to harvest and preserve

Simply grow your plant until they are mature. You will be able to see that they are by the way the leaves grow.

When they are fully developed and a uniform color, they are ready. Simply take your gardening scissors and snip off the leaves right at the base where they grow onto the stem.

Make sure you do not harm the stem as you work.

Lay them out on a paper towel to dry, or speed the process in a food dehydrator. When they are completely dried out, scoop the leaves into a small glass jar with an airtight lid until you are ready to use them.

Uses:

A wide array of uses come with this lovely mint. Use for aches and sores, headaches, stomach aches, or any other joint pain.

Spearmint

How to grow

Place in a pot and leave in direct sunlight, water daily.

How to harvest and preserve

Simply grow your plant until they are mature. You will be able to see that they are by the way the leaves grow.

When they are fully developed and a uniform color, they are ready. Simply take your gardening scissors and snip off the leaves right at the base where they grow onto the stem.

Make sure you do not harm the stem as you work.

Lay them out on a paper towel to dry, or speed the process in a food dehydrator. When they are completely dried out, scoop the leaves into a small glass jar with an airtight lid until you are ready to use them.

Uses:

Use to flavor meats and savory dishes, teas, and medicinally for aches and pains.

Lemon Mint

How to grow

Place in a pot and leave in direct sunlight, water daily.

How to harvest and preserve

Simply grow your plant until they are mature. You will be able to see that they are by the way the leaves grow.

When they are fully developed and a uniform color, they are ready. Simply take your gardening scissors and snip off the leaves right at the base where they grow onto the stem.

Make sure you do not harm the stem as you work.

Lay them out on a paper towel to dry, or speed the process in a food dehydrator. When they are completely dried out, scoop the leaves into a small glass jar with an airtight lid until you are ready to use them.

Uses:

Use to flavor meats and savory dishes, teas, and medicinally for aches and pains.

Apple Mint

How to grow

Place in a pot and leave in direct sunlight, water daily.

How to harvest and preserve

Simply grow your plant until they are mature. You will be able to see that they are by the way the leaves grow.

When they are fully developed and a uniform color, they are ready. Simply take your gardening scissors and snip off the leaves right at the base where they grow onto the stem.

Make sure you do not harm the stem as you work.

Lay them out on a paper towel to dry, or speed the process in a food dehydrator. When they are completely dried out, scoop the leaves into a small glass jar with an airtight lid until you are ready to use them.

Uses:

Use to flavor meats and savory dishes, teas, and medicinally for aches and pains.

Chocolate Mint

How to grow

Place in a pot and leave in direct sunlight, water daily.

How to harvest and preserve

Simply grow your plant until they are mature. You will be able to see that they are by the way the leaves grow.

When they are fully developed and a uniform color, they are ready. Simply take your gardening scissors and snip off the leaves right at the base where they grow onto the stem.

Make sure you do not harm the stem as you work.

Lay them out on a paper towel to dry, or speed the process in a food dehydrator. When they are completely dried out, scoop the leaves into a small glass jar with an airtight lid until you are ready to use them.

Uses:

Use to flavor meats and savory dishes, teas, and medicinally for aches and pains.

Chapter 14 – The Best of the Rest

Tarragon

How to grow

Plant seeds roughly ½ inch into the soil, and space them 1 inch apart. Set in a well lit area and water frequently.

How to harvest and preserve

Simply grow your plant until they are mature. You will be able to see that they are by the way the leaves grow.

When they are fully developed and a uniform color, they are ready. Simply take your gardening scissors and snip off the leaves right at the base where they grow onto the stem.

Make sure you do not harm the stem as you work.

Lay them out on a paper towel to dry, or speed the process in a food dehydrator. When they are completely dried out, scoop the leaves into a small glass jar with an airtight lid until you are ready to use them.

Uses:

Another essential herb for your blood. This is the herb to turn to for heart health. You will find that it lowers your blood pressure, evens out your blood sugar, and it helps prevent blood clots.

An all in one herb for perfection.

Sage

How to grow

Plant seeds roughly ½ inch into the soil, and space them 1 inch apart. Set in a well lit area and water frequently.

How to harvest and preserve

Simply grow your plant until they are mature. You will be able to see that they are by the way the leaves grow.

When they are fully developed and a uniform color, they are ready. Simply take your gardening scissors and snip off the leaves right at the base where they grow onto the stem.

Make sure you do not harm the stem as you work.

Lay them out on a paper towel to dry, or speed the process in a food dehydrator. When they are completely dried out, scoop the leaves into a small glass jar with an airtight lid until you are ready to use them.

Uses:

Sage is excellent for the digestive tract. Take it and promote a healthy gut.

Marigold

How to grow

Plant seeds roughly ½ inch into the soil, and space them 1 inch apart. Set in a well lit area and water frequently.

How to harvest and preserve

Simply grow your plant until they are mature. You will be able to see that they are by the way the leaves grow.

When they are fully developed and a uniform color, they are ready. Simply take your gardening scissors and snip off the leaves right at the base where they grow onto the stem.

Make sure you do not harm the stem as you work.

Lay them out on a paper towel to dry, or speed the process in a food dehydrator. When they are completely dried out, scoop the leaves into a small glass jar with an airtight lid until you are ready to use them.

Uses:

Marigold has been used as an anti-inflammatory as well as a relief for stomach pain. Keep it on hand for a variety of ailments.

Feverfew

How to grow

Plant seeds roughly ½ inch into the soil, and space them 1 inch apart. Set in a well lit area and water frequently.

How to harvest and preserve

Simply grow your plant until they are mature. You will be able to see that they are by the way the leaves grow.

When they are fully developed and a uniform color, they are ready. Simply take your gardening scissors and snip off the leaves right at the base where they grow onto the stem.

Make sure you do not harm the stem as you work.

Lay them out on a paper towel to dry, or speed the process in a food dehydrator. When they are completely dried out, scoop the leaves into a small glass jar with an airtight lid until you are ready to use them.

Uses:

An herb used to treat headaches and joint pain, this is the herb to have on hand if you work with your hands often. It is going to ease a lot of the pain without all of the side effects of synthetic medication.

Chamomile

How to grow

Plant seeds roughly ½ inch into the soil, and space them 1 inch apart. Set in a well lit area and water frequently.

How to harvest and preserve

Simply grow your plant until they are mature. You will be able to see that they are by the way the leaves grow.

When they are fully developed and a uniform color, they are ready. Simply take your gardening scissors and snip off the leaves right at the base where they grow onto the stem.

Make sure you do not harm the stem as you work.

Lay them out on a paper towel to dry, or speed the process in a food dehydrator. When they are completely dried out, scoop the leaves into a small glass jar with an airtight lid until you are ready to use them.

Uses:

Welcome relaxation into your life when you indulge in this rich herb. Perfect to chill out even the most stressful day.

Chapter 15: Herbal Antibiotics for your Allergies

Allergies are quite a common occurrence today and their frequency are only increasing. Food allergies are in abundance and pet allergies leave people in hives, even worse that this the confluence of hot weather and pollen leave thousands of allergy suffers struggling to breathe every year. Is there anyway we can counteract the effects of these bothersome allergies?

As it so happens, there are several completely natural, herbal remedies that can reduce or even completely eliminate much of these allergy systems. Amazingly, even though allergies are a reaction to the natural environment, herbs produced from that same troublesome environment are fully capable of counteracting their effect! Check out some of the best herbal allergy fighters out there.

Nettle Leaf

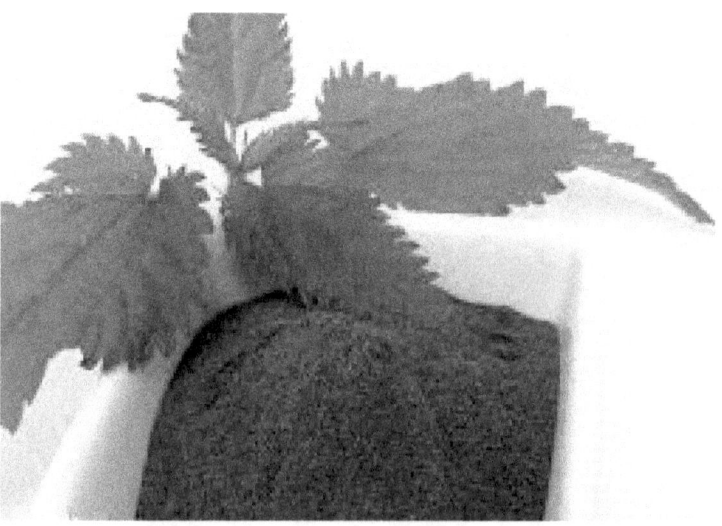

Are your allergies making you swell up like a balloon and causing your nose and eyes to water like faucets? Then you should look into administering some Nettle

Leaf. Because this herb is not only a strong antibiotic, it is also a strong antihistamine that can effectively block adverse reactions your body might have to certain elements of the environment. Nettle leaf grows rather abundantly in many locations and can be ground up into a fine powder that can be applied directly to the skin. If you start to feel your allergies kicking in later this spring, you should keep some nettle leaf in quick supply.

Local Honey

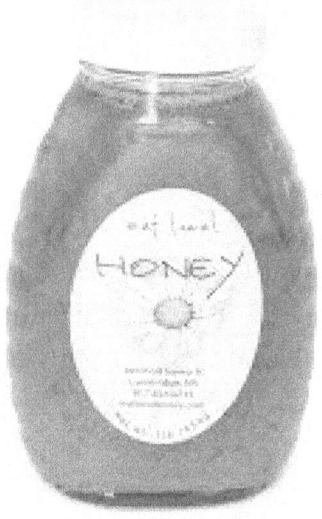

Believe it or not, local honor from your region can work essentially like an allergy shot. Amazingly, while that honey is being produced by the bee, it is being inundated with special protective features very specific to that region. Regularly consuming the honey locally produced with from where you live can greatly boost your ability to fight off the same allergies that your local stomping grounds produces! More importantly, the pollen the bee ingested during its production of the honey should help get your body better used to the local pollen of the area and not react so badly to it. This kind of locally made honey should be available at your local farmer's markets and during the spring and summer you may find them well stocked by local street vendors as well.

Butterbur

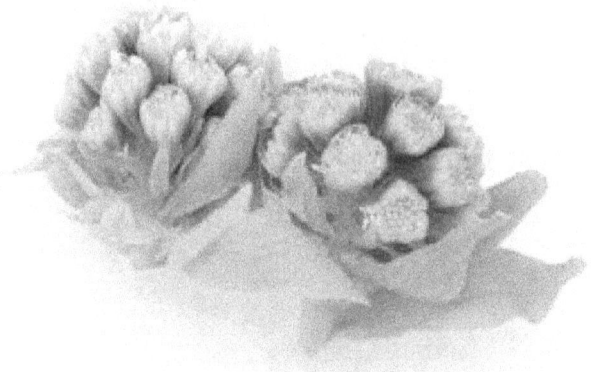

If you suffer every time pollen season comes around, using Butterbur as a natural herbal remedy can greatly alleviate your symptoms. Butterbur also works as an antihistamine for runny noses. Best of all this is an herbal treatment for pollen allergies that won't dope you up and make you sleepy! Feel free to take this herbal antibiotic allergy fighter as much as needed. Butterbur has also been known to provide relief to migraine headache sufferers. So if you have ever had a bad headache or bad allergies, butterbur is worth your attention. Just grind this herbal antibiotic down into a fine, dusty powder and serve it in a soothing tea. You will be feeling better in no time.

Turmeric

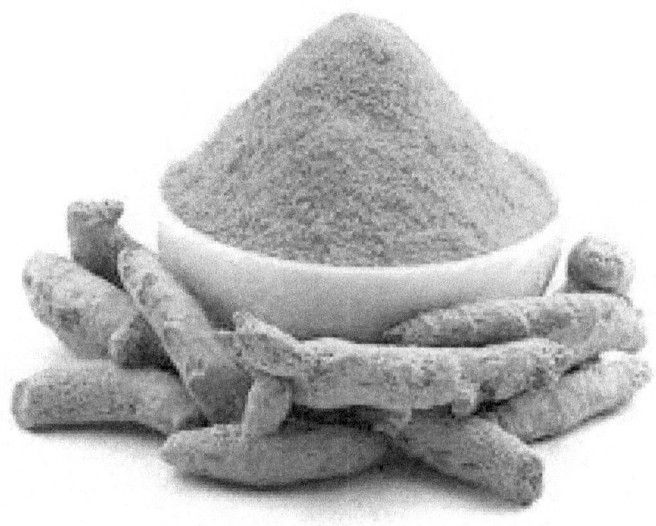

This spicy herb that is so often used to spice up curry and rice, can also be used to take a dent in your allergies! Turmeric works well as a nasal decongestant clearing up runny nasal passages. It also seems to be able to ward off colds completely if taken on a regular basis. The secret ingredient in Turmeric that works so well to fight allergies is called "curccumin". This special additive seems to work just as well as many over the counter drugs when it comes to stifling the cold and allergy season. So instead of going to your doctor and getting him to write another prescription, you should go to your health food store and get a healthy dose of Turmeric!

Milk Thistle

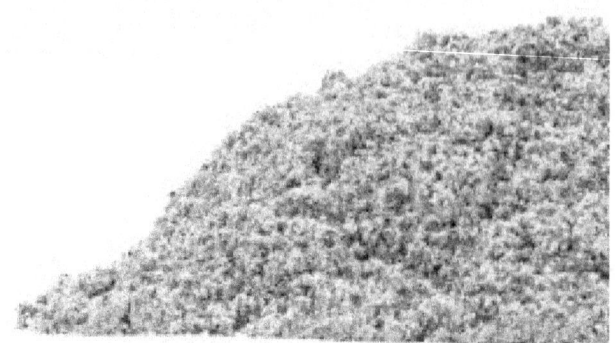

Milk Thistle is a great antibiotic herb to have when it comes to reducing allergy related inflammation and other histamine reactions to allergies. Milk Thistle also provides a great boost to liver function. This herb is able to treat several liver ailments such as jaundice, hepatitis, and even cirrhosis. Milk Thistle has also been known to greatly lower cholesterol. But it is its prevention of seasonal allergies that Milk Thistle is best known for, so when that pollen count begins to rise during the change of season, be sure to have a batch of milk thistle on hand! Milk Thistle can be boiled in teas or applied directly to the skin. Use this wonder herb as much as needed!

Red Clover

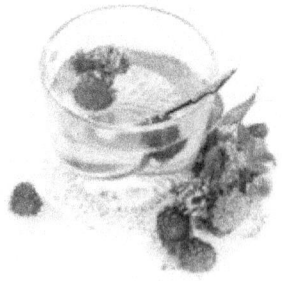

This herb is another well known allergy resistance booster. It boosts the immune system and even boosts the body's red blood cell count. Red clover works to improve cardiovascular health while it fights off allergens in the environment. Red Clover also thins the blood and prevents blood clots. It is rather amazing that this dark red clover is so beneficial to the red blooded human being, but whether you are having a severe allergy outbreak or just need to strengthen your cardiovascular health, red clover has something for you. Just grind this herb up and either sprinkle it over your food or boil it in a nice glass of tea.

Yarrow

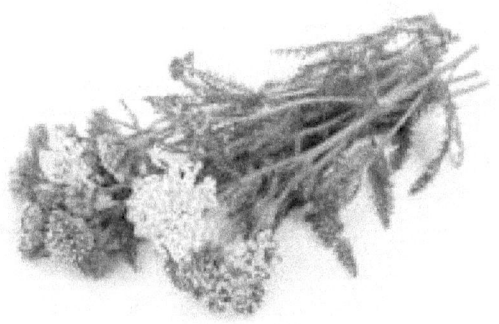

This herb helps to eliminate allergy related congestion, the ingredients in this herb work to quickly dry out the sinus greatly improving runny nose, coughing, and the like. But much more than this, if you are ever left inured with a severe cut, this herbal antibiotic can stop the bleeding almost instantaneously. Yarrow is a fast acting antibacterial, antiseptic. Yarrow has also been known to promote bile production in the gallbladder which is an essential treatment in some allergic reactions. This herb works great when ground into a fine powder and either ingested or applied directly to your skin.

Guduchi

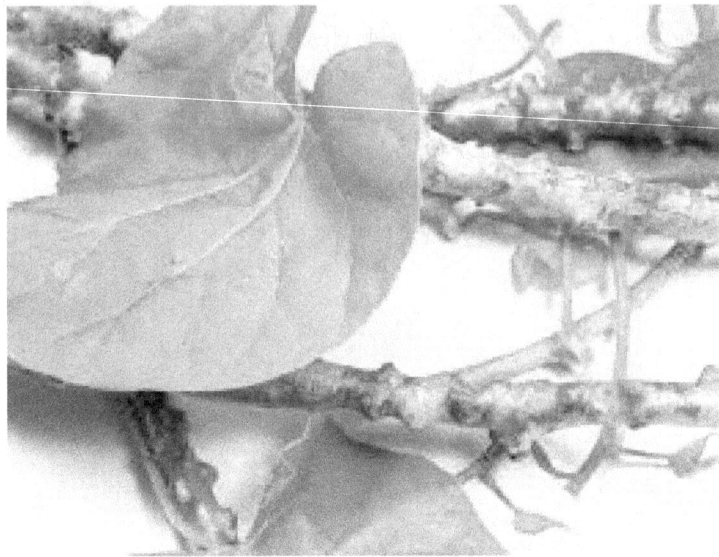

Used for thousands of years in Ayurvedic medicine, this herb can be used to relieve inflammation brought on by allergies. This antibiotic herb is also fully capable of boosting the immune system, clearing up skin conditions, and even relieving hay fever. Guduchi is well worth a try during the allergy season. Guduchi is quite effective in relieving common allergic symptoms such as sneezing and a runny nose. Guduchi also helps in a wide range of stomach problems such as nausea, cramps, and even colitis. Guduchi is an allergy fighter with a lot of inborn benefits. Guduchi can be delivered in a variety of ways; it can be either ingested, or massaged into the skin as oil, for immediate affect.

Spirulina

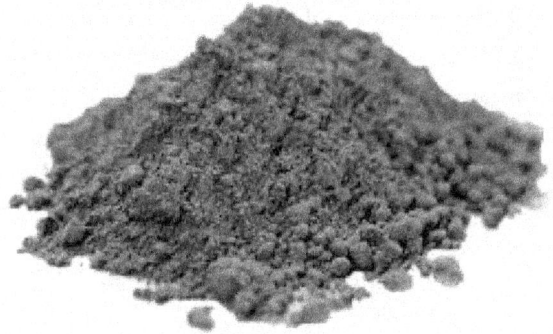

This antibiotic herb packs a vitamin B12 punch and when it is ground down into a fine powder and administered to allergy sufferers it has been proven to greatly improve nasal congestion. Spirulina is actually an algae and one of the best ways to take Spirulina is to boil the herb in water and then serve it up in a nice hot glass of tea. You can also ground Spirulina into powder and sprinkle it over your food. Spirulina also boosts the immune system and enhances the production of your body's cells, allowing tissue to heal much faster. You've got yourself a great bargain when you get a hold of some good Spirulina.

Horseradish

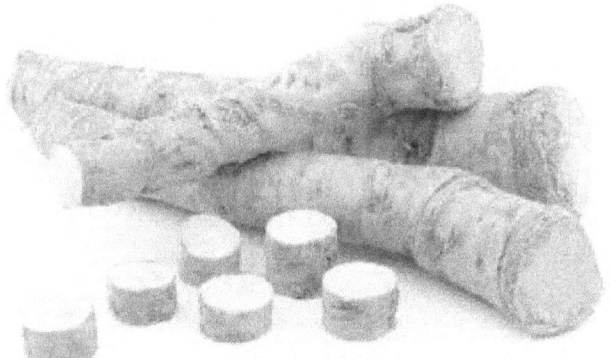

Horseradish is not just good as a sandwich condiment it is also a good way to get rid of a congested sinus! In fact, the dreaded sinus infection doesn't stand a chance against a small dash of horseradish! Believe it or not, along with breaking up congestion brought on by allergies, this tangy herb has even been known to help people smile! That's right, horseradish increases blood flow to the face, and even stimulates the facial muscles responsible for that lovely grin on your face! That's why I always smile when I go to Arby's because those guys have quite a monopoly on their horsey sauce!

Ginkgo

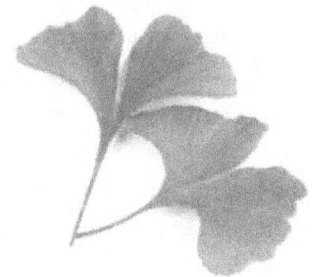

This herbal antibiotic is also an antihistamine allergy blocker. Ginkgo has many different beneficial chemical compounds within it, all of which act as natural anti-inflammatory agents. Not only that, ginkgo improves the flow of oxygen to the brain, helping to aid memory and other cognitive function. As an allergy fighter however, ginkgo is absolutely superb in battling sinusitis. If you are feeling at all under the weather, don't hesitate to try out some ginkgo. Ginkgo can be found at most health food stores and vitamin shops.

Chapter 16: The Antibiotic Properties of these Healing Herbs

Of course when you have a book titled, "Herbal Antibiotics" you are going to want to discuss the main lifeblood of these plants, and that is their antibiotic properties. Here are some of the best antibiotic features that these herbs can provide for you.

Anise

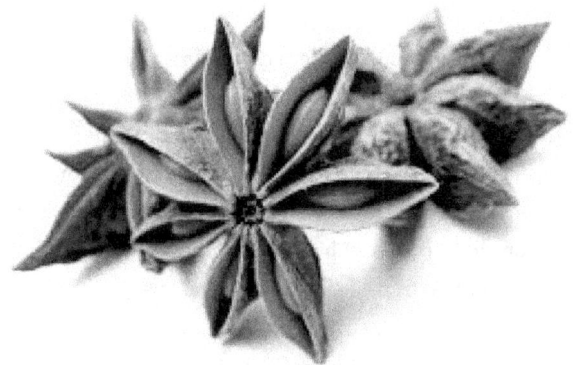

This herb is a familiar ingredient to those who prepare East Asian cuisine, but it also happens to be one of the best bacteria fighting herbs you can find with a ton of helpful antioxidants to boot! Anise is also a natural diuretic that works to clear out and cleanse the kidneys and colon, detoxifying the entire body from its routine use. This antibiotic herb has also been known to help those with breathing problems by expanding the lungs. Grind it in powder, boil it's leaves or eat it raw, any way you look at it, this herb has some seriously powerful antibiotic properties!

Basil

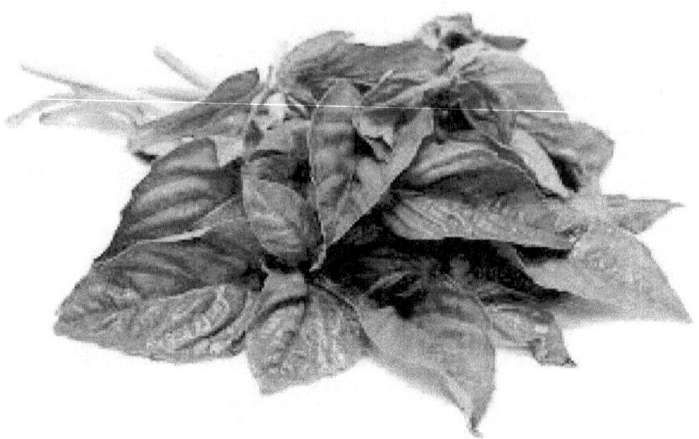

Another often used ingredient in food, this herb also disinfects like there is no tomorrow! Basil kills bacteria on contact! Basil helps to ward off the common cold and is a great treatment for breathing disorders such as bronchitis. Basil is also good for the hearth and has been rated as one of the best herbs for cardio-vascular health. This refreshing herb has a way of recalibrating the entire body. These are all good reasons to give this antibiotic healing herb a try. Basil is best administered in powdered form or by boiling the leaves in water.

Bay Leaf

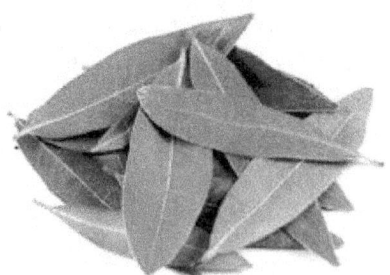

A common item in many kitchens, Bay Leaf is well known for its extra healing properties, helping everything from acne to stomach pain. The oil from Bay Leaf also destroys harmful bacteria and greatly reducing its ability to grow in the future. Bay Leaf has also been known to reduce many kinds of fungi, so if there are any bacteria or fungus among us, just get out some Bay Leaf and you can make some short work of it! Bay leaves are also good for your digestive health, cleansing your system and clearing up stubborn indigestion. This herb makes a trip to the health food store well worth it!

Chervil

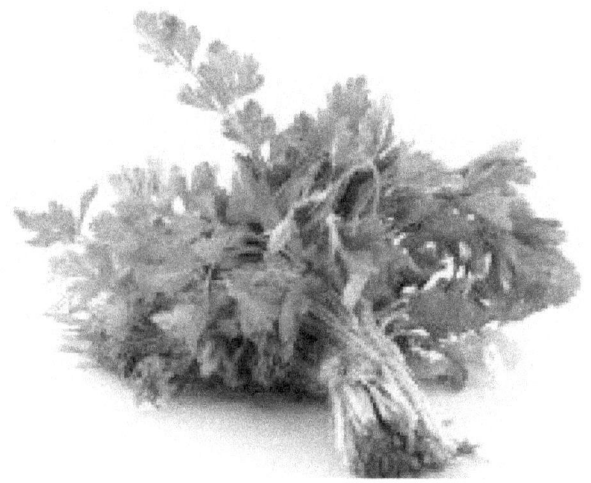

Chervil is another great herbal antibiotic that gets its bacteria fighting power from its leaves. When these leaves are ground down into a powder and mixed into tea, this concoction can be drunk to eliminate chronic coughs and ease feverish states. Chervil also works as a soothing sleep aid helping you get the rest that you need. Amazingly some even claim, even though there is no scientific research to back it up, that Chervil actually increases the likelihood of having good dreams! So if you've been plagued by nightmares, scare that bogeyman right out the door with some Chervil! Chervil also relieves headaches and calms upset stomachs, you should sleep well with some chervil at your side!

Cloves

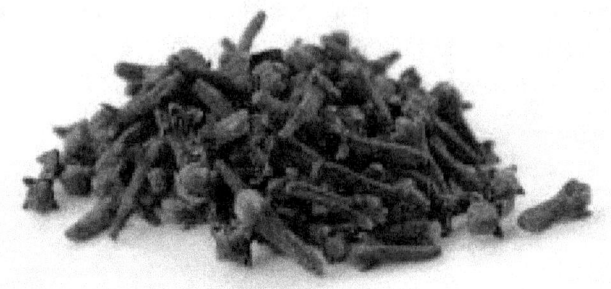

An antibiotic herb used by ancient dentists of the bygone past, it has long been known that placing boiled cloves to the teeth and gums can eliminate bacteria and prevent harmful inflammation. Cloves also work as a mild anesthetic, reducing any pain that you feel. This herb also does well to treat the flu and fight colds. In addition to all of these benefits, cloves also work exceedingly well as a food preservative. Cloves are commonly available at most health food stores, vitamin shops, and even at your local grocery.

Cumin

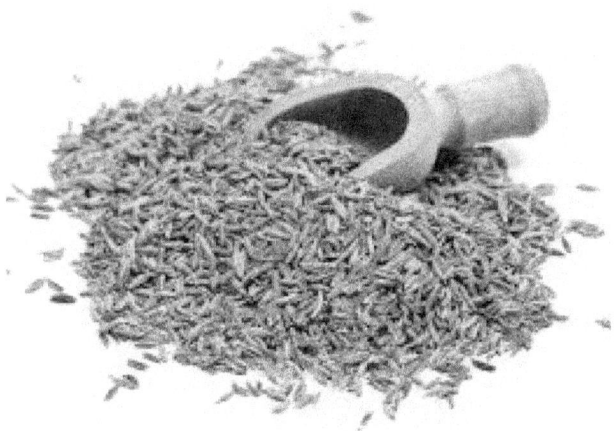

Cumin is not only a good herbal antibiotic in its own right, it also aids and enhances any prescription antibiotics that you may already be taking. Just put some cumin powder in your food and you will see the effects immediately as this herb goes the distance protecting you from harmful bacteria. Cumin also works great as a bronchodilator, working as a treatment for asthma and other inflammatory conditions of the lung. Cumin is a refreshing and invigorating herb. And to top it all off this herbal antibiotic also cures anemia! You've just got to try it!

Dill

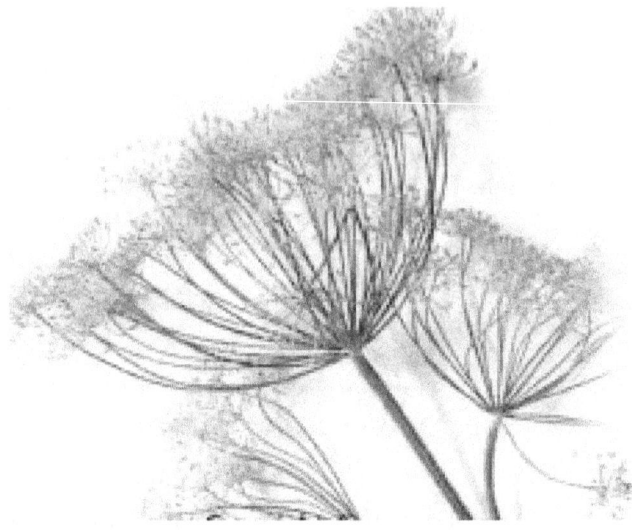

Dill is a little known but wonderful herbal antibiotic that has a powerful ability to fight off infections. Dill can be harvested the easiest in the summer and early fall months of the year. Just grind this herb into powder and either apply it direct to the skin or sprinkle it over your favorite food. As well as its antibiotic properties dill has many other benefits such as treating heartburn, indigestion, and even the hiccups! I can personally attest to the hiccup part. I once had a bout of hiccups that was so frustrating I called into work! I added some dill to my tea that morning however, and it made short work of those unwelcome interruptions. A little bit of dill is always good to have around!

Marjoram

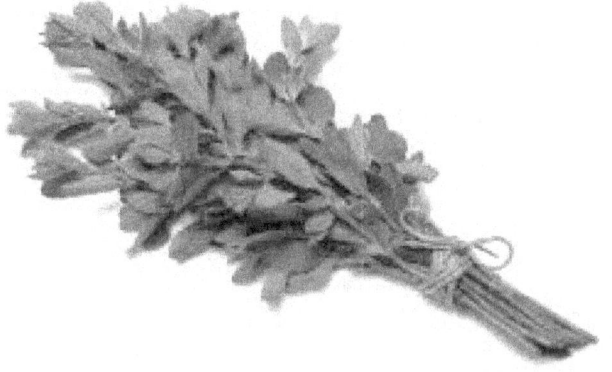

This herb's antibiotic properties serve it well as a cold fighter and fever reducer. Marjoram helps to eliminate infections caused by both bacteria and viruses. Usually administered through the oil extracted from its leaves, this herb can be applied directly to the skin. Marjoram leaves are also of great benefit when they are boiled in tea, helping to ease sore throats and even the most stubborn of coughs. This herb also helps to relieve intestinal bloating and is a great antioxidant. Use as needed and this herbal antibiotic will do the trick!

Mustard Seed

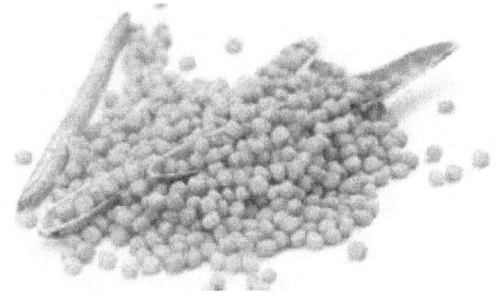

Many benefits can be derived from this herb, such as relief from cramps, inflammation, arthritis, and muscle pain just to name a few. But right along with all of these great attributes, much can be also said about Mustard Seed's great properties as an herbal antibiotic. Mustard fights off bacterial infections upon contact and works wonders against the common cold. Mustard is also good for cardiovascular health and stimulates circulation in the body. Who would have thought something you normally slap on a hotdog could be so healthy? Try this herb today for a healing and enriching experience.

Oregano

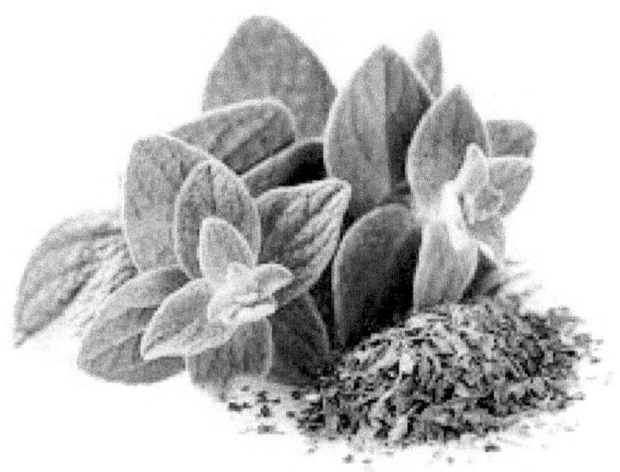

You may already be familiar with this herb as an additive to your lasagna, but it also has quite a few awesome attributes as an antibiotic. Through the oil extracted from Oregano seeds, Parsley has the power to fight off bad infections from both bacteria and fungus. Even Athlete's foot has been treated with Oregano. Urinary tract infections have been eliminated with this herb and kidney stones have been reduced in severity from Oregano's antibacterial properties. Oregano busts up colds and gets rid of jaundice. These are just some of the main cures Oregano provides, look into it a bit further and you will no doubt discover many more uses from this wonder herb! Always keep a good amount of this herbal antibiotic in stock!

Tarragon

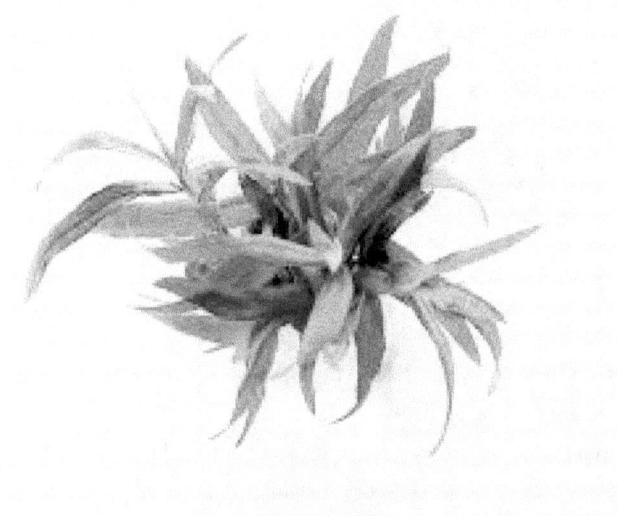

This is a natural antibiotic that can be used to counteract the effects of food poisoning and other bacterial infections. Tarragon is so potent yet palatable it was even once used as a food preservative to extend the expiration date on many different dishes. Tarragon also helps treat insomnia. The best way to take Tarragon is as a powder either sprinkled over your food or boiled in a nice glass of hot tea. Another aspect of Tarragon as an herbal health aid, is its ability to stimulate appetite in cancer patients. Tarragon has helped others in so many ways; you shouldn't hesitate to try it for yourself. Get some quality Tarragon today!

Thyme

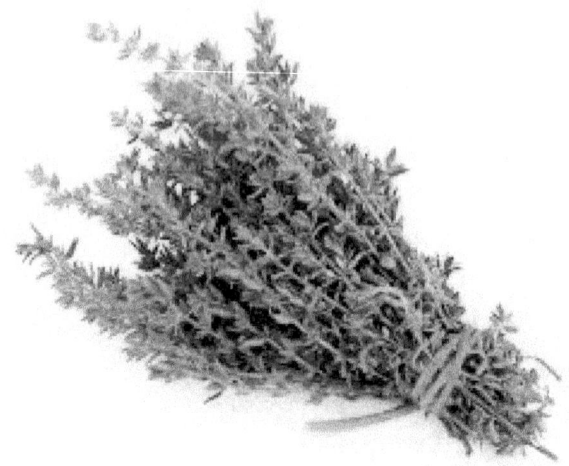

This antibacterial herb is a great tool to use to prevent the spread of bacteria in meat when you are cooking food. Just sprinkle some Thyme in your pan and you can rest assured that it will be working to protect your food from harmful bacteria. Thyme is also good for chronic dry coughing. I personally used to have a problem of getting a bad cough every winter, but after I started taking some Thyme, that cough all but disappeared.

Thyme, when boiled down in hot tea, has a wonderful way of soothing a throat. It is even effective in treating laryngitis and other bacterial infections of the throat. Thyme works well to reduce inflammation and also works as a dietary aid against upset stomach and indigestion. This is an all around great herbal antibiotic to have around for any occasion that may present itself.

Coriander

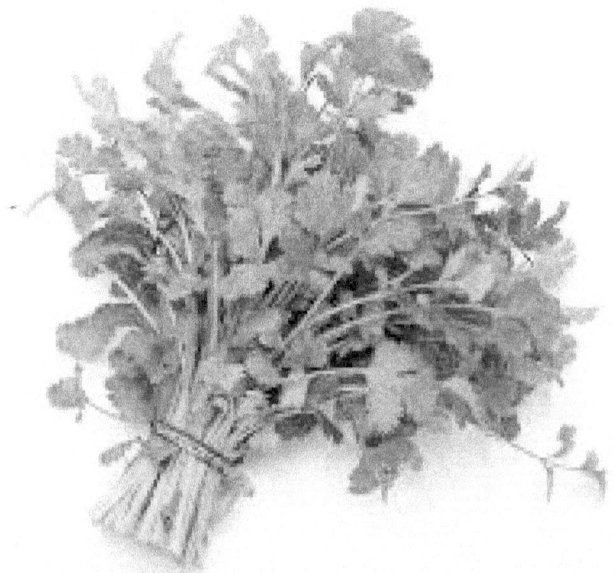

Coriander is yet another good choice when it comes to an herbal antibiotic that can work to prevent food poisoning. There are also many kinds of infections—infections that resist even prescription antibiotics—that can be successfully treated with a good batch of coriander. This herb is also good for the joints. Just apply it directly to the skin and inflammation will go down. Other extra healing attributes associated with this herbal antibiotic is its ability to get rid of hemorrhoids, and even increase the production of milk for pregnant women. Coriander is quite a multitasking herb don't hesitate to use it.

Fennel

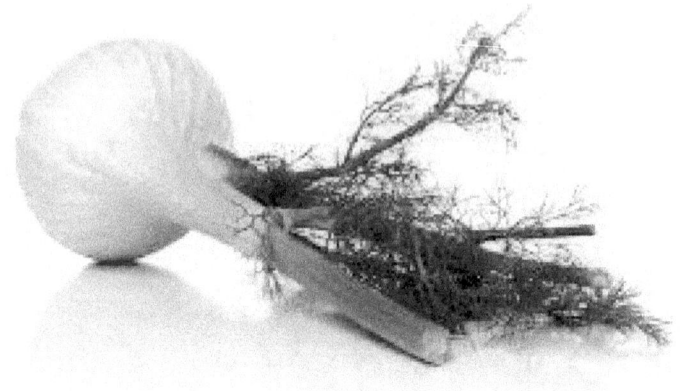

This herb works as a strong antibacterial and antifungal aid. Just grind it into a powder and add it to your food or skin in order to receive treatment from this powerful herb. As an added bonus fennel has also been known to boost the user's metabolism. This herbal antibiotic is commonly used in order to decrease discomfort associated with bloating, cramps and other typical stomach problems. If you are feeling under the weather, you should try out fennel immediately, you won't be disappointed.

Lemon Balm

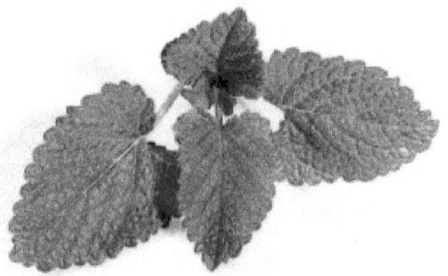

Lemon is a natural disinfectant, so much so that we have by popular demand, lemon scented dish soap, lemon scented air fresheners, and a wide variety of other lemon based disinfectants. Even if the "lemon scent" is an artificial additive, the well known concept of lemon's natural cleaning and disinfecting ability is ingrained in the consciousness. This is no different with lemon balm. This herb is about as antibacterial as it gets, and instant contact with lemon balm stops bacteria in its tracks. This herb is best taken as a hot tea made with its dried out leaves. As well as disinfecting, lemon balm is quite capable of soothing your throat and calming your nerves as well. So whether you need a bacterial disinfectant or just a good cup of relaxing tea, lemon balm is well worth your time and effort.

Nutmeg

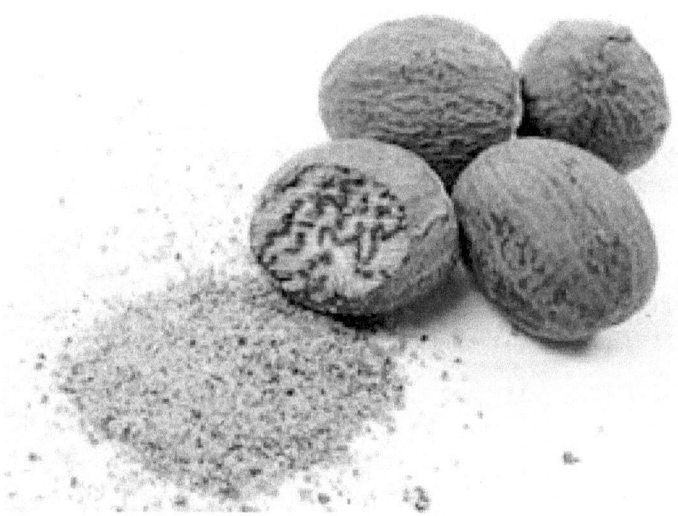

This is one of my favorite herbs, it goes great with dessert, but it also goes great as an herbal antibiotic. Nutmeg is actually highly effective against one of the worst bacterial outbreaks to plague mankind; E. coli. Yes, that's right, the dreaded Ecoli, and even staph infections are no match for trusty old nutmeg. Nutmeg has also been known to fight off cold sores, and reduce the effects of arthritis and joint pain; just rub this herb right onto the skin and you will start feeling the effects almost immediately.

Sage

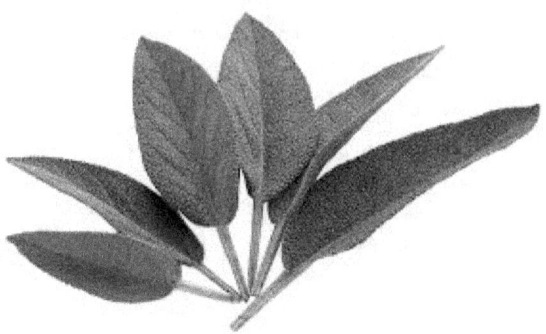

Already known to reduce inflammation, Sage is also a wonderful way to fight off bacteria. The leaves are usually boiled in tea to create a soothing tonic that can soothe throats and ease stomach pain. Sage has also been reported to treat everything from Alzheimer's disease to diabetes with regular administration. One healing property for this antibiotic herb that I can personally vouch for is its ability to help asthma. Having suffered from breathing problems most of my life, I can attest that just breathing in the aroma of sage can do well to open up even the most constricted of airways. All of these herbs have antibacterial properties and then some!

Chapter 17: Precautions to Use Herbal Medicine

To begin with, herbal medicines are used by multiple people which the following purposes:

- Anti-microbial

- Anti-bacterial

- Iodine wash

- Anti-viral

Every measurement of anti-biotic should be weighed deliberately, since re-supply won't come, in the lack of supplies decent homemade information may spare the life of somebody you adore.

Nonetheless, it is important that given the sheer number of home grown meds, and impressive heterogeneity inside and between brands, it is not possible to assess all items for their pharmacology. Albeit some natural pharmaceuticals have had broad examination, a large portion of them have not. Indeed, even those that have been moderately very much concentrated frequently have little data in extraordinary populaces, for example, pediatric, pregnant or lactating ladies, or geriatric populaces, and subsequently, alert ought to be utilized while prescribing natural medications to these populaces.

Some of the side effects of using peppers survival medicine are as follows:

1. Skin allergies:

Topical home grown antifungal and antibacterial operators, for example, tea tree oil and lavender are capable of causing rashes or skin disturbance, particularly if utilized at full quality. Before utilizing any topical home grown item, attempt a skin patch test. Place a little measure of the item within the elbow on one arm as it were. Hold up a couple days. On the off chance that the range stays clear, continue with utilizing the home grown item

2. Dizziness:

Everybody's body is distinctive, and some individuals are more delicate to herbs than other individuals. Herbs used to treat uneasiness, melancholy and a sleeping disorder may bring about extreme daytime lethargy in specific people. These herbs incorporate chamomile, valerian and kava, with valerian and kava being the in all probability offenders. Abstain from driving or utilizing apparatus until you're certain of the impacts of the herb.

3. Photosensitivity:

People taking herbal medicines treat despondency or uneasiness may discover their skin turning out to be more delicate to the sun. They may blaze all the more effortlessly. Commonly, reasonable haired and light-cleaned Caucasians have the most astounding occurrence of photosensitivity, yet this home grown reaction is thankfully uncommon. Common instances of photosensitivity happen when individuals take high dosages of herbal medicine, or take it over a drawn out stretch of time. In the case of taking herbal medicine, maintain a strategic distance from an excess of sun presentation

However, if someone desires to eliminate the danger of getting harmed by using dangerous herbs or plants as medicines, then he must adopt following precautionary measures:

Learn to differentiate between harmful and harmless plants:

Firstly, one must learn how to differentiate between those plants which are harmful and which one of them are harmless. This very approach will help the person choosing the plants for medicinal purposes. If a person is unaware about the plants, then he might get confused and use a wrong herb. This can cause various allergies and can even lead to death

1. Never utilize any plant without the validness of its character:

Secondly, any plant must not be utilized before its complete recognizable proof. This may represent a risk to one's wellbeing. Hence, a plant must not be utilized before its 100% distinguishing proof

2. Do not get confused between plants:

Thirdly, multiple plants look similar to one another. However, not all of them are useable. Therefore, never get confused by the deceiving looks of the plant

3. Avoid excessive use of the herbs:

Fourthly, one should avoid the excessive use of plants and herbs. If one uses the herb in an excessive quantity, then it might cause damage to the person using the herb. In the event that you utilize home grown supplements, take after mark guidelines deliberately and utilize the endorsed dose as it were. Never surpass the suggested dose, and search out data about who ought not to take the supplement.

4. Look for reactions:

If any symptoms, for example, sickness, unsteadiness, cerebral pain, or furious stomach, happen, diminish the measurements or quit taking the home grown supplement

5. Be ready for an unfavorably responses:

A serious hypersensitive response can bring about trouble relaxing. If any unlikely event occurs, rush to the emergency to avoid any harm.

6. Do some research:

Research about the organization whose herbs you are taking. All home grown supplements are not made equivalent, and it is best to pick a respectable maker.

Moreover, following things must be checked before using any homemade medicine:

- Has the manufacturer put some effort in developing the herbal product or if he is employing the some one's research.

- Does the item make abnormal or difficult to demonstrate claims?

- Does the item mark give data about the institutionalized equation, reactions, fixings, bearings, and safeguards?

- Is the provided data clear and simple to peruse?

Conclusion: An Extra Helping

Infections produced by bacteria are becoming increasingly common. We live in a bubble of contamination, with sick people and compromised immune systems. And once you get just the *wrong kind* of combination of weakened antibodies and bacterial assailants, you could find yourself becoming very ill, very fast. These severe kinds of infections have a hard time getting better on their own. These are the ones that usually make you head into the clinic so your doctor can prescribe you a heavy dose of antibiotics.

But these self same antibiotics have become quite a problem in their own right. I'm sure you have heard the latest reports from your nightly news broadcast over the epidemic of people being overprescribed antibiotic medication? Well, due to this overuse of prescription antibiotics, the bacteria (smart little guys) have learned to adapt and overcome the typical pharmaceutical treatment! This has laid to strains of superbugs that are not so easily controlled, as they were in the past.

Since the doctor's prescription has since fallen short of the mark, many now, more than ever, have begun to turn their attention to herbal treatment. Because even though these bacteria bugs have learned to outsmart the synthetic creations of man, they can't escape nature, and simple herbs like nutmeg can have these nasty critters on the run once again.

I predict that soon the whole medical profession will wise up to this fact and begin stocking up their clinics with antibacterial herbs as a frontline defense. Until then take what you have learned in this book to heart, and keep yourself safe and healthy with an extra helping of herbal antibiotics!

FREE Bonus Reminder

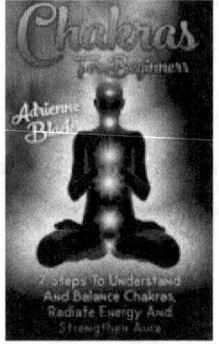

If you have not grabbed it yet, please go ahead and download your special bonus E book *"Chakras for Beginners. 7 Steps To Understand And Balance Chakras, Radiate Energy, And Strengthen Aura"*.

Simply Click the Button Below

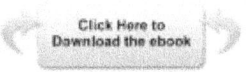

OR Go to This Page

http://lifehacksworld.com/free

BONUS #2: More Free & Discounted Books & Products

Do you want to receive more Free/Discounted Books or Products?

We have a mailing list where we send out our new Books or Products when they go free or with a discount on Amazon. Click on the link below to sign up for Free & Discount Book & Product Promotions.

=> **Sign Up for Free & Discount Book & Product Promotions** <=

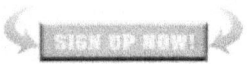

OR Go to this URL

http://zbit.ly/1WBb1Ek